Situational Judgement Test
for the Foundation Years Programme

Dr Omar Taha

Dr Mizanul Hoque

Dr Belinda Kessel

First Edition 2012
Second Edition 2013

British Library Cataloguing in Publication Data
A catalogue record for this book is available from the British Library.

ISBN: 978-1492918264

Copyediting by Editorial Consultant, Cherry Mosteshar of The Oxford Editors
Book typesetting, formatting and design by Mahir Arzoky
CreateSpace, North Charleston, South Carolina

Acknowledgements

We would like to formally acknowledge the following individuals who contributed full scenarios (questions + explanations) as well as innovative ideas to the book:

Dr Abid Shoaib, MBBS BMedSci, GP VTS
Dr Mark Toynbee MBBS MA MBioch, SHO
Dr Mohammad Mahmud MBBS BSc, Core Medical Trainee
Dr Tomide Isinkaye MBBS BSc, Academic FY2
Dr Imran Yasin Siddiq MBBS BMedSci, GP VTS
Dr Sumit Sinha-Roy, MBChB BSc, Core Medical Trainee
Mr Christopher Buckle MRCS BSc MFMLM, Core Surgical Trainee
Dr Mohammed Razwan Ashiq MBBS BSc, GP VTS
Dr Samia Nesar MBBS, GP VTS
Dr Inderpreet Kaur Dhaliwal MBBS, FY2
Dr Marcela Schilderman MBBS BSc, Psychiatry SpR
Dr Sam Chabuk MBBS BSc, GP VTS
Dr Phuong Thao Nguyen MBBS MA, FY2
Dr Harriette May Packer MBChB, FY2
Dr JFW Ndikum MBBS BSc, SHO
Dr Lucia Anthonypillai MBBS BMedSci, GP VTS
Dr Jonathan Anthonypillai MBBS BSc, FY2
Dr Ary Phaily MBBS, FY2
Dr Maeve Gallagher MBcHB, FY2
Dr Shalini Fernando MBChB, SHO

We would like to formally acknowledge the following individuals who were part of the official Appraisal Group for the book. This group was involved in reviewing and critiquing the questions and their respective explanations and rationale, all of which was considered to produce the final formulation of the questions seen in this book:

Senior Appraisers
Dr Mark Toynbee MBBS MA MBioch, SHO
Dr Tomide Isinkaye MBBS BSc, Academic FY2
Dr Sumit Sinha-Roy MBChB BSc, Core Medical Trainee
Dr Mohammad Mahmud MBBS BSc, Core Medical Trainee
Dr Abid Shoaib MBBS BMedSci, GP VTS
Dr Imran Yasin Siddiq MBBS BMedSci, GP VTS

Dr Mohammed Razwan Ashiq MBBS BSc, GP VTS
Dr Nafis Hossein MBBS BSc, GP VTS
Dr Raphael Teatino MBBS BSc, GP VTS
Dr Kevin Kelleher, Deputy Postgraduate Dean for Secondary Care &
Consultant Geriatrician
Dr Gloria Yu, Consultant Stroke Physician & Former Associate
Clinical Director
Mr Mohamed Y Hammadeh, Foundation Programme Training
Director & Consultant Urologist
Dr Mukhtarul Islam, General Practitioner
Mr Muhilan Pathmamohan BSc MSc LLB, Medical Lawyer

General Appraisers
Dr Rula Najim MBBS BSc DMCC MRCP, Clinical Oncology SpR
Dr Mohammed Owais Rahman MBBS BSc, GP VTS
Dr Jonathan Anthonypillai MBBS BSc, FY2
Dr Hafiz Uddin MBBS BSc, Clinical Teaching Fellow
Dr Rumman Ahmed MBBS BSc, Radiology SpR
Dr Zaiba Hashmi MBBS, SHO
Dr Asad S Mahmood MBBS BSc, FY2
Dr Zeeshaan Hasan MBBS BSc, FY2
Dr Madiha Hussain MBBS BSc, FY2
Dr Mohammed Monem MBBS BSc, FY2
Dr Yayganeh Chiang MBBS BSc, FY2
Dr Salmaan Saleem MBBS BSc, FY2
Dr Rana Najim MBBS BSc, GPVTS
Dr Sabrina Quereshi MBBS BSc, FY2
Dr Muhammad Liyawdeen MBBS BSc, FY2
Dr Bhupinder Singh Hoonjan MBBS BSc, FY2
Dr Suleman Kanani MBBS BSc, FY2
Dr Mohammed Fozlul Kadir MBBS BSc MSc, FY2
Dr Muhammad Patel MBBS, FY2
Dr Hichem Ben Hamida MBBS BSc, FY2

A special thank you to *Sameehah Ahmed* **for her administrative support**

Foreword

The inception of the Foundation Programme in the United Kingdom in 2005, was a key moment in the history of training of junior doctors in the UK. The foundation programme has ensured that junior doctors working in the UK are trained according to a clear curriculum and within parameters of a specific structure, which includes appropriate supervision and training.

Central to the foundation programme, have been the generic skills required of a fully functional doctor of medicine. These include more than just the technical skills or indeed the academic knowledge, but the skills that enable doctors to function effectively, safely and humanly. The methods used to appoint applicants to the foundation programme have evolved over the last seven years, and a key component to this process has been a means of measuring a medical student's competence in relation to these generic skills.

Up and until 2011, these generic skills were assessed on the basis of five white space questions, for which each applicant had up to two weeks to formulate an appropriate answer. While this method has been able to distinguish applicants, it has been recognised as having significant deficiencies. It is because of this that the Medical School's Council, the Department of Health together with the UKFPO have introduced the situational judgement test (SJTs) as the chosen method to measure the aptitude of aspiring foundations doctors.

This book provides an opportunity for aspiring foundation applicants to both practice SJTs and understand the skills that may be required of them as they embark on their future medical career, and this will be welcomed by the applicants to the programme.

Dr. Andrew Frankel
Postgraduate Dean for Health Education
Lead for London Foundation Training

Contents

Background to the Foundation Programme 1
What are Situational Judgement Tests? 1
How Situational Judgement Tests are assessed 3
About this book 4
Clarification of terms 6
Some advice to get you started 6
About the authors 8
Practice Paper 1 Questions 11
   Question 1: Home time! 12
   Question 2: Hospital or hotel? 13
   Question 3: Cremation Form 14
   Question 4: Yellow card, surely? 15
   Question 5: Medical students arrive for teaching 16
   Question 6: Nobody has to know? 17
   Question 7: An ideal catch – I think I've found 'the one' 18
   Question 8: Up to mischief 19
   Question 9: A case of child abuse 20
   Question 10: Family pressure 21
   Question 11: A flexible what? 22
   Question 12: Feedback to the boss! 23
   Question 13: I want my name on the audit 24
   Question 14: Suspecting a colleague of stealing 25
   Question 15: Providing medical advice to a colleague 26
   Question 16: Prescribing practices 27
   Question 17: Unwritten drug chart 28
   Question 18: Self-discharge 29
   Question 19: Sick leave 30
   Question 20: An angry pharmacist 31
   Question 21: You want my honest opinion? 32
   Question 22: Capacity versus confidentiality? 33
   Question 23: A laxative mistake 34
   Question 24: Ditched by your SHO 35
   Question 25: Challenging the SHO's decision? 36
   Question 26: Ward round prescribing 37

Question 27: On call and unresponsive! 38
Question 28: The 'crash-call' relative 39
Question 29: Prioritising your workload 40
Question 30: The battle for annual leave 41
Practice Paper 1 Answers.. 42
Practice Paper 2 Questions.. 98
Question 1: Just hours before the operation begins 99
Question 2: Nutritional treatment over medications 100
Question 3: Nobody likes a bully...................................... 101
Question 4: Anxious relatives 102
Question 5: The referral bleep 103
Question 6: Second Opinion 104
Question 7: Off home at five on the dot............................. 105
Question 8: Third year wrestles with a cannula 106
Question 9: ABG from the wrong patient!.......................... 107
Question 10: A Stressed SHO 108
Question 11: Doctor in the family...................................... 109
Question 12: The cannula in a cardiac arrest 110
Question 13: The difficult arterial blood gas 111
Question 14: Coping with a heavy workload....................... 112
Question 15: Fatal potassium levels................................... 113
Question 16: The fitting patient 114
Question 17: A Distressed Family 115
Question 18: A Consultant's Complaint 116
Question 19: Colleague calling in 'sick' 117
Question 20: In need of handwriting lessons 118
Question 21: The sandwich.. 119
Question 22: What are the results of my scan doctor?........... 120
Question 23: Drop in saturations 121
Question 24: Locum here for a laugh.................................. 122
Question 25: First time procedure....................................... 123
Question 26: Only the best doctor will do 124
Question 27: Caring for colleagues..................................... 125
Question 28: Nightmare cannula... 126
Question 29: Disinterested Medical Student........................ 127
Question 30: A possible mishap.. 128
Practice Paper 2 Answers.. 129

Practice Paper 3 Questions.. **185**

Question 1: Wedding day... 186

Question 2: Reversing the Liverpool Care Pathway?............ 187

Question 3: You made the nurse cry............................. 188

Question 4: Wrong dose and the patient has gone home........ 189

Question 5: Racial abuse on the ward........................... 190

Question 6: Family kept waiting................................ 191

Question 7: Attending your prize award ceremony............... 192

Question 8: Skiving off the post take round.................... 193

Question 9: Can't get work off my mind........................ 194

Question 10: Too many referrals!................................ 195

Question 11: Just trying to relax with your flatmates........... 196

Question 12: Final year student lets slip....................... 197

Question 13: Colleague gone AWOL............................ 198

Question 14: Patient fed up and wants to go home.............. 199

Question 15: FY2 intruding..................................... 200

Question 16: Reprimanded for minor error...................... 201

Question 17: A kind gesture.................................... 202

Question 18: All I'm asking for is to go to theatres............. 203

Question 19: Parents will 'have a go'........................... 204

Question 20: Squeamish patient & the blood cultures.......... 205

Question 21: Dealing with death................................ 206

Question 22: Lazy colleague.................................... 207

Question 23: Heartbroken....................................... 208

Question 24: 'It's a free country'............................... 209

Question 25: You lose your cool at the nurse................... 210

Question 26: Doctor, She's turned red.......................... 211

Question 27: The rush to discharge............................. 212

Question 28: No harm in exaggerating?......................... 213

Question 29: Jehovah's Witness and blood transfusions........ 214

Question 30: Compulsory FY1 teaching dilemma............... 215

Practice Paper 3 Answers.. **216**

Background to the Foundation Programme

An elaborate process aimed at improving selection to the Foundation Programme has led to significant changes being made to the Foundation Programme application process, one of the major changes being the replacement of the 'white space questions' by Situational Judgement Tests (SJTs). SJTs were found to have a greater level of reliability and validity, thus distinguish between candidates more effectively, and to assess a broader skill and competency base. They were also seen to be more sustainable and cost effective. The Foundation Programme application process combines the applicant's academic achievements and their score on the SJT paper, an invigilated examination performed in a time-restricted environment, to determine allocation to Foundation Year Programmes.

What are Situational Judgement Tests?

SJTs will be an assessment modality that is new to most medical students. SJTs assess the response of candidates to a wide range of possible scenarios that they can be expected to face in their work as a junior doctor. This format of assessment tests a wide range of skills, experiential knowledge base and personality traits. The effectiveness of SJTs has been supported by research evidence and has been demonstrated by its popular use in various business and civil recruitment processes, including recruitment to General Practice training.

Studies have been carried out to highlight the main attributes that are expected from a foundation year doctor. These core attributes are as follows:

- Commitment to professionalism
- Coping with pressure
- Effective communication
- Learning and Professional Development
- Organisation and planning
- Patient Focus
- Problem solving and decision-making
- Self-awareness and insight
- Working effectively as part of a team

See www.isfp.org.uk for further details on these attributes.

The SJT examination will have a broad range of questions that will seek to assess all the aforementioned competencies.

The SJT questions for the Foundation Programme are currently of two formats. The first of these format types includes a scenario followed by five possible responses, where candidates are required to rank all five options in order of appropriateness, from one to five; where the first option is assumed to be the most appropriate response and the fifth being the least. It is important to mention that all five options may be viable or non-viable choices to make in reality, however, it is the relative difference between them that the candidate must identify and prioritise. An example of this question format is as follows:

Home time!

You are preparing to go home at the end of your long day shift, and on your way out you go to an outlier ward to return a pen torch that you had used that day. The nurse whose torch you borrowed approaches you and tells you that she's been waiting for a doctor who promised to come up 30 minutes ago to prescribe a patient some PRN (as required) Ibuprofen as he's recently been having some pain. She asks you if you could just sign this on the drug chart.

Rank in order *the following actions in response to this situation (1= Most appropriate; 5= Least appropriate)*

a) Sign the drug chart and thank the nurse for the pen torch
b) Inform the nurse your shift has finished but offer the bleep number of the next doctor on shift
c) Ignore the nurse's request and tell her your shift has finished
d) Refuse to sign and inform her that the other doctor knows the patient better
e) Return the pen torch, inform the nurse to file a complaint against the doctor, then leave

The second question format follows a similar concept, however, there are eight options from which three are to be chosen, without the need to rank them:

You want my honest opinion?

A group of medical students have come for some clinical skills teaching as their final exams are a few months away. You happen to have a very pleasant patient who consents to being examined - a lower limb neurological examination. The student who examines the patient is nervous and only remembers to test light touch and proprioception; his examination technique is also poor. At the end of the session, the student brings his logbook for a signature under 'performed a peripheral neurological examination'.

*Choose the **THREE most appropriate** actions to take in this situation*

a) Inform the student that you will sign on this occasion, however, he needs to improve, and thus should come back next week and perform the examination again

b) Advise the student that he might fail his finals if he doesn't revise his clinical skills and refuse to sign

c) Sign his logbook as a confidence building measure and comment that he 'wasn't too bad but can improve'

d) Ask him to come back later this week and perform the examination again for the signature

e) Encourage him to reflect on his examination and refuse to sign

f) Hold a democratic vote amongst the on-looking colleagues as to whether he deserves the signature

g) Sit with the student in a quiet room and ask him to talk you through the peripheral lower limb examination for the signature

h) Offer him material to read up on but don't sign

How Situational Judgement Tests are assessed

It is important to realise that for many scenarios, there is often no 'absolutely correct answer', as individuals have different ways of doing things and thus there may be small variations in responses. The marking does take this fact into account and marks are allocated based on how close one's answer is to the 'model answer'. This means that 'near misses' will also result in the candidate acquiring marks. The ranked questions require more thought and take longer to answer, and thus, have a greater share of points. There is no negative marking, however, if a candidate ties two answer options (e.g. two separate answers are both ranked as being second best), he or she receives zero marks for each of the tied options. If a candidate selects more than three options for the multiple-choice questions, a mark of zero is given for the entire question.

Currently, each ranking SJT question is allocated a maximum of 20 marks, a maximum of 4 marks per correct answer. This is allocated based on how close the respondent's answer compares with the model answer.

For the multiple choice SJTs, four marks were given for each correct answer, enabling a maximum of 12 marks per item.

Please see www.ifsp.org.uk for more details on the scoring convention and for general SJT format and structure, which is prone to modifications each year.

About this book

As has been mentioned, most students will be unfamiliar with SJTs and thus it is important for candidates to sit the SJT exam with a clear understanding of what SJTs are and how best to approach them.

Thus, the fundamental aims of this book are to:

- ❖ Explain what SJTs are and how best to approach them
- ❖ Help increase familiarity with SJT question formats, and to obtain practice in answering questions within timed settings
- ❖ Provide thorough explanations of the answers
- ❖ Highlight key educational elements within the explanations that will help build the reader's knowledge and skills in answering SJTs

The questions have been tailored to meet the format and style of the SJT exam. A combination of five-option and eight-option scenarios is included, with a split of two-thirds and one-third respectively, in line with the current exam format. The questions have been divided into three papers, with the aim that should students wish to test themselves, they can allocate one hour per paper, with an average rate of two minutes per question being in alignment with the SJT exam.

The answers aim to provide thorough explanations using current guidelines where appropriate (specifically from the General Medical Council's (GMC) Good Medical Practice guidance and The New Doctor, as well as from other supplementary guidelines). We have ensured that this second edition of the book corresponds to the latest Good Medical Practice guidelines issued by the GMC in 2013. Some explanations also include further teaching points to help you gain a further understanding of the competency being tested, as well as to familiarise yourself with basic principles that will prove indispensible for the SJT paper as well as your work as a Foundation Year Doctor.

A rigorous process was implemented when designing and appraising the SJTs presented in this book to maximise the reliability and validity of each individual question. This book contains a wide range of SJT scenarios to ensure that all the core Foundation Programme competencies are comprehensively covered. The questions and answers brought together the experiences of over 50 doctors from varying levels and specialities, including multiple Foundation Programme Directors, to ensure that the scenarios and their responses were valid, and relevant to the SJT exam and Foundation Programme curriculum. The book also involved professionals with backgrounds inclusive of medical law, medical ethics, psychology and medical education to sew together realistic and challenging scenarios with valuable learning points for the exam as well as working life. Many of the junior doctors who participated in the design of this book had firsthand experience of the National SJT Pilot Exam, and thus provided a unique insight into question format, style and design. Each question was appraised by multiple assessors to gauge:

> How realistic the scenario was and it's level of clarity
> Concurrence with the answers
> Clarity of explanations and agreement with the rationale behind the explanations
> An overall appraisal of each question and whether it is answerable within 2 minutes

The questions were also piloted amongst a further selected group of Foundation Year 2 doctors, and a good level of concurrence for the correct answers to each question was established.

Clarification of terms

Throughout the book the terms 'House Officer' and 'Foundation Year 1' have been used interchangeably as in accordance with current practice within hospitals, as many of the senior colleagues still tend to use the older name (House Officer). Similarly, the term 'Senior House Officer (SHO)' is also used interchangeably with 'Foundation Year 2'. However, it is worth mentioning that those previously known as SHO also included doctors who, in line with the current system, are within their Core Training years, just before Registrar level. Some scenarios mention 'on-calls' which, as you have not started working yet, may be difficult to fully appreciate. To help you to have a better understanding of the scenarios in which you are described as being 'on-call', a brief explanation is provided here: The on-call FY1 works as a member of the on-call team who are either covering emergency admissions primarily from the A&E department, or they are covering the acute needs of the inpatients when the regular team is not present (evenings, nights and weekends). When working in A&E (referred to as '1st on-call' or 'admitting on-call' at some trusts), the FY1 is allocated a patient whom they clerk in, initiate a basic plan where appropriate and discuss the patient with a senior. This role may be performed at anytime of the week - day or night. The FY1 who covers the ward patients (sometimes called '2nd on-call' or 'ward cover') is usually handed over tasks to perform by the day team and is also called by nurses to address other patient needs that may arise (e.g. an unwell patient).

Some advice to get you started

Like every exam, it is vital to make good preparation and obtain practice in answering questions in a time-controlled environment. It is worthwhile noting that the SJT paper does not assess clinical knowledge. The following advice will help optimise your ability to effectively answer SJTs.

✓ Remember that it is your competencies to be an effective FY1 that is being assessed. These competencies are laid out in the

GMC's Good Medical Practice and the Foundation School Person Specification. It is absolutely vital that you familiarise yourselves with both these documents. Other GMC guidance, including 'The New Doctor', can also prove helpful in answering the SJTs.

✓ When answering questions, do not make any assumptions. It is vital that you only use the information that has been provided to you. Read the question and each answer option before you start answering the SJT.

✓ Good time management is key to performing well, so time yourself when sitting these practice papers, and do not spend more than one hour per paper. That gives you two minutes per question on average, the same rate that you would be given in the actual exam.

✓ When reading through a question, think about the core competencies that the question is seeking to assess (for example, is the scenario concerned with patient care as the primary focus? Or teamwork, or probity...? – it can be a combination of more than one core competency). That will help you think back to principles you have learnt pertaining to the respective competencies being assessed and help identify the most appropriate responses.

✓ The answer options that you are provided with for a given scenario need to be looked at relative to the other answer options in the same scenario. All the possible options may be very good or very poor, it is about distinguishing between them and identifying the best ones.

✓ In many SJT questions you will be able to identify the 'very correct' and/or 'very incorrect' answer options quite easily. Realising this will make it easier to focus your attention on the answer options that are less clearly distinguishable, and will help you save time.

✓ It is important to understand that for the 'rank 5' questions, each answer option is to be taken on its own merit. So once you have selected one option as being most appropriate, you should ignore that and re-assess each of the remaining options alone against the scenario, as if re-answering the question again. Be careful not to fall into the trap of ranking answers that you feel would follow the previous action consecutively – you'll lose precious marks! Rather, you should select one answer, and then ignore it from the remaining options, and answer the question again according to which of the remaining options you think would be most appropriate.

✓ For the 'select 3' questions make sure that your answers do not contradict in any way, and that the answers work well together. Contrary to the 'rank 5' questions, the 'select 3' options are not mutually exclusive and should be taken together with each other to form the most appropriate response to the scenario.

✓ There is no negative marking, so answer all questions (however, be careful not to answer more than three options for the multiple choice exam, otherwise a mark of zero will be allocated for that question).

✓ In the exam, be very careful that you have correctly transcribed all answers to the mark sheet.

We hope you enjoy working through this book as much as we enjoyed compiling it. We are confident that this book will be a very useful tool in helping you prepare for your SJT paper and your future practice as a junior doctor. Finally, we wish you all the best for the Foundation School Application and your final year at medical school.

Omar Taha
Mizanul Hoque
Belinda Kessel

We'd be delighted to hear from you. If you have any comments or feedback about *SJT for the Foundation Years Programme*, please contact us at info@medgrad.org.uk.

About the authors

Dr. Omar Taha (BSc MBBS) – Foundation Year 2 Doctor (Studied BSc in Psychology)

Omar Taha is a Foundation Year 2 doctor in the South Thames Foundation School, having graduated in July 2012 with a distinction in clinical practice. He has participated in piloting the National SJT Exam and has been certified for involvement in SJT item development. Omar has published and presented his research work at national and international levels, and was presented the Merit Award by the South Thames Foundation School for his contribution to Teaching.

Dr. Mizanul Hoque (BSc MBBS) – GP VTS
(Studied BSc in Medical Education)

Mizanul Hoque is a GP VTS in the London Deanery. He graduated in July 2011 with distinctions in medical sciences and clinical practice. He was awarded *proxime accessit* for the University of London Gold Medal Award. Mizanul has a 1st class BSc Hons in Medical Education, and has been involved in various research projects in education, presenting some of his research work at national and international conferences. He was presented the Merit Award for Excellence in Foundation Programme by Health Education London.

Dr. Belinda Kessel MB ChB, MSc (Clinical Gerentology), FRCP –
Consultant Physician and Geriatrician; Foundation Training
Programme Director (KHT)

Belinda Kessel is a Consultant in General and Elderly Medicine with a Special Interest in Movement Disorders and works at the Princess Royal University Hospital, part of Kings' Healthcare Trust, a role she has had since 2001. She has extensive experience in education and is a mentor to medical students and clinicians. She acts as a GKT Tutor for fourth year medical students as well as a supervisor for fifth year medical students. Belinda is also a clinical and educational supervisor for doctors of all grades including foundation years, a role where she ensures adequate clinical, academic and personal development. She has been Foundation Training Programme Director at the Kings' Healthcare Trust since the inception of the Foundation Programme. In this role, she is responsible for the delivery and implementation of the training programme for all foundation year doctors at the trust. She works closely with junior doctors and is responsible for signing off each one after ensuring the successful achievement of the required competencies, as outlined in the Foundation Programme curriculum and GMC guidelines.

Practice Paper
1
Questions

Question 1: Home time!

You are preparing to go home at the end of your long day shift, and on your way out you go to an outlier ward to return a pen torch that you had used that day. The nurse whose torch you borrowed approaches you and tells you that she's been waiting for a doctor who promised to come up 30 minutes ago to prescribe a patient some PRN (as required) Ibuprofen as he's recently been having some pain. She asks you if you could just sign this on the drug chart.

Rank in order *the following actions in response to this situation (1= Most appropriate; 5= Least appropriate)*

a) Sign the drug chart and thank the nurse for the pen torch

b) Inform the nurse your shift has finished but offer the bleep number for the next doctor on shift

c) Ignore the nurse's request and tell her your shift has finished

d) Refuse to sign and inform her that the other doctor knows the patient better

e) Return the pen torch, advise the nurse to file a complaint against the doctor, then leave

Question 2: Hospital or hotel?

This is the fifth time in the past month that Mr. Wernicke has come into hospital with an episode of alcohol withdrawal. He is feeling a bit shaky and confused and is now sitting on the ward floor being provocative towards the other patients, demanding his lunch and in clinical need of Chlordiazepoxide. You have spoken to him each time about his alcohol abuse but he hasn't taken notice and refuses to go to any support groups. Rather, he enjoys the food and comfort provided at the hospital and is happy to stay in this 'hotel'.

Rank in order *the following actions in response to this situation (1= Most appropriate; 5= Least appropriate)*

a) Explain to him that if he continues to misbehave you will have to call security

b) Inform him that he needs to sign up for an alcohol support service to improve his behaviour

c) Ignore him for the time being as this should act as behavioural conditioning for his demeanour and repetitive admissions

d) Ask him to sit on his chair, prescribe him his Chlordiazepoxide and ask the nurse to bring his lunch

e) Discuss the situation with social services

Question 3: Cremation Form

One of the patients on your Care of the Elderly ward has just passed away and you have confirmed the death. You broke the news to a family member 15 minutes ago who thanked you for your help, and informed you that they plan to cremate the body as soon as possible based on family tradition. You sign the Certification of Death form and have now been asked by the bereavement team to complete the cremation form. Problematically, you have a personal objection to cremation based on your own family tradition and prefer not to sign.

Rank in order the following actions in response to this situation (1= Most appropriate; 5= Least appropriate)

a) Apologise and explain to the family member that you will be unable to sign the form but another colleague can

b) Sign the form reluctantly

c) Ask one of your medical colleagues who has seen the body to sign the form instead

d) Offer alternative avenues the family may wish to explore other than cremating the body

e) Arrange a date to discuss the situation with your clinical supervisor

Question 4: Yellow card, surely?

A patient came in earlier today with cellulitis having injected heroin into her groin. She was given Benzylpenicillin and Flucloxacillin, but unfortunately she developed a severe and rare reaction to the drugs, despite the notes clearly stating that she has *'No Known Drug Allergies'* along with patient testimony. She is now stable on the ward but is quite traumatised by the whole ordeal.

Rank in order *the following actions in response to this situation (1= Most appropriate; 5= Least appropriate)*

a) Sit with her and listen to her concerns and fears

b) Ask the ward pharmacist to give you an overview on drug reactions

c) File a complaint against the doctor who prescribed the penicillin

d) Send a report to the Medicines and Healthcare products Regulatory Agency and let her know how to do the same

e) Take a minute out to call your friends and say that you'll be late for the planned football match tonight

Question 5: Medical students arrive for teaching

While on the ward, a group of eager looking third year medical students arrive for their first day of clinical attachments and introduce themselves to you. You are tied up with various jobs on the unusually busy ward and have a list of bloods to take. You rationalise that this could be an opportunity for teaching as well as help in reducing your current blood-taking work load.

Rank in order the following actions in response to this situation (1= Most appropriate; 5= Least appropriate)

a) Give a brief overview of venepuncture, delegate the students a patient each, and tell them to report back to you once they're done taking blood

b) Ask the students to write down the steps of venepuncture as a group, whilst you collect the equipment, and then to observe you

c) Go with them and supervise each one as they attempt to take blood

d) Ask the students to accompany you on your jobs and to just observe

e) Refer the students over to the doctors' mess to find a colleague who is free and can teach them

Question 6: Nobody has to know?

Mrs Liston came in earlier today with sharp right-sided pleuritic chest pain and abdominal discomfort, and she was diagnosed with a pulmonary embolism. On taking routine investigations you find her β-HCG levels to be positive. You disclose the results of the tests to Mrs Liston and ask whether she knew that she was pregnant, to which she nods her head and says *'nobody has to know'*. Despite best efforts to manage her condition, she passes away that evening. The family arrive at the hospital distraught, and the husband approaches you asking *'what could have caused this?'*

Rank in order *the following actions in response to this situation (1= Most appropriate; 5= Least appropriate)*

a) Inform him that the exact cause of death isn't clear and this condition can occur spontaneously which may be the case with his wife

b) Take him into a quiet room and explain to him honestly that her pregnancy may have been the underlying reason for her death

c) Inform him that it is too early to be sure and a post-mortem may be required, but you will inform a senior to sit down and speak to him soon

d) Take a brief sexual history from him and ascertain from his knowledge whether there was a chance that Mrs Liston could have been pregnant

e) Explain to him that you have a suspicion, however, you can't be sure until you have discussed it with your seniors

Question 7: An ideal catch – I think I've found 'the one'

Miss Parker, a 22 year old woman, was admitted last week with a severe bout of ulcerative colitis and has been recovering on the ward ever since. During your ward rounds, she has been making suggestive comments towards you, and has made you feel uncomfortable when around her, so much so that you almost forgot to take blood from her this morning. After returning to take blood however, she asks whether you are single and whether you would be interested in going on a date. This proposition has not been made to any of the seniors on your team. The SHO has remarked that she'd be an ideal catch for you, and you confess an interest in her.

Rank in order *the following actions in response to this situation (1= Most appropriate; 5= Least appropriate)*

a) Inform Miss Parker that you need time to think about it, however, you might be interested in her offer

b) Inform Miss Parker that your primary aim is to get her feeling better and out of hospital, after this is achieved you can discuss the matter further

c) Explain to Miss Parker that her comments have been completely inappropriate and that you have no interest in dating anyone right now, then leave and take a minute to think about the situation

d) Decline the offer and inform a senior that you no longer feel comfortable with her behaviour and suggest whether it would be better to hand the patient over to the team on the other half of the ward

e) Smile at Miss Parker and crack a joke, then carry on with your jobs on the ward

Question 8: Up to mischief

Whilst away with your mates on a trip to The Lake District, you are questioned by the police for being rowdy outside the museum. To your misfortune, the police also find a stash of cannabis in your pocket which they confiscate and give you a warning for. Your friend points out that at least you didn't get 'nicked' for being anti-social like you had only last month back in South London.

Rank in order the following actions in response to this situation *(1= Most appropriate; 5= Least appropriate)*

a) Count your lucky stars and stay on your best behaviour for the rest of the trip

b) Phone up the GMC and tell them what just happened as well as last month's incident

c) Seek advice from your defence body in case it affects your GMC registration

d) Turn over a new leaf and sell the rest of the cannabis you had saved in the flat

e) Carry out an internet search just to make sure this doesn't affect your medical profession

Question 9: A case of child abuse

You are the surgical house officer on-call. Your team has admitted a 14 year old girl with suspected appendicitis. While you are taking her history she reveals that her father has been physically abusing her at home but she does not want anybody to know.

Rank in order the following actions in response to this situation (1= Most appropriate; 5= Least appropriate)

a) Try to convince her to let you get help for her but assure her you will not tell anyone if she does not want you to

b) Call the social services team

c) Call the police

d) Discuss the case with your seniors/senior nursing staff

e) Get a collateral history from the girl's father

Question 10: Family pressure

You see an elderly patient in pre-assessment clinic for an elective left hemicolectomy for colonic adenocarcinoma. She confides in you that the situation is all too much for her to cope with. She says that she does not want to go ahead with the surgery and just wants to be left alone to die peacefully. She tells you she feels pressured by her family to go through with the surgery.

Rank in order *the following actions in response to this situation (1= Most appropriate; 5= Least appropriate)*

a) Ask the patient if she has expressed these thoughts to anyone else and explore her feelings further

b) Tell her not to worry, the team will look after her and things will be ok

c) Tell her you will cancel her operation and you can refer her to the MacMillan nursing team

d) Empathise with her thoughts and explain you will inform your consultant

e) Tell the patient you will ask one of the specialist cancer nurses to come and talk to her about these concerns

Question 11: A flexible what?

During a busy post-take round, you see a patient with your registrar. She is a 44 year old South Asian lady admitted with PR bleeding. She does not speak fluent English. Your registrar explains to the patient that he would like to book a flexible sigmoidoscopy to investigate the cause of the bleeding. The patient nods her head and the registrar hands you the request form to take down to endoscopy. You do not feel the patient fully understood what the registrar was saying nor the details of the proposed procedure.

Rank in order the following actions in response to this situation *(1= Most appropriate; 5= Least appropriate)*

a) Drop the form off to endoscopy and try to re-consent the patient after the round

b) Drop the form off to endoscopy without trying to re-consent as this procedure is being done in the patient's best interests

c) Speak to your registrar about your concerns over the patient's understanding of what was said

d) Speak to the nurse in charge and request a translator for the patient

e) Fill out the request form but hold on to it until you feel the patient fully understands the proposed procedure

Question 12: Feedback to the boss!

You are near the end of your FY1 medical placement and your consultant has requested formal feedback online within an appraisal form. You have had a lot of difficulty working with your consultant. In your view, she has been indecisive and not clear about care plans. She has continually asked you to meet up to review all the patients on the ward after your normal working hours. You also find her doctor-patient manner patronising. However, you have not mentioned this before and you are aware that the consultant is your clinical supervisor who needs to sign you off. You are worried that if you mention your concerns in the feedback, the consultant will be able to trace the comments as you are the only junior doctor on the team.

Rank in order the following actions in response to this situation *(1= Most appropriate; 5= Least appropriate)*

a) Appreciate that you are a junior and therefore try to make your comments inoffensive and toned down, while still attempting to convey most of your views across

b) Avoid completing the feedback form in case it will affect your working relationship and discuss your concerns with your educational supervisor instead

c) Complete the feedback form accurately describing all the areas of concern you have where appropriate, even if you know this may count badly against you in future forms and references

d) Before completing the form, discuss your concerns with other colleagues in the mess to ensure that this is not only your view and/or a misunderstanding

e) Complete the form in a positive way that will hopefully reflect in your own feedback from the consultant

Question 13: I want my name on the audit

You and your SHO discuss possible areas of improvement on the ward and develop an idea for an audit you think will be interesting and help inform changes to improve patient care. You discuss it with your consultant who approves the idea and you both undertake the work over several evenings and weekends. The day before you are due to present the results at the hospital grand round, your registrar informs you that he needs an audit for his portfolio and asks you to put his name on the audit as well.

Rank in order *the following actions in response to this situation (1= Most appropriate; 5= Least appropriate)*

a) Decline, as the registrar has not made a contribution to the work so it would be unethical

b) Decline but offer to help him on another joint audit

c) Put the registrar's name on the presentation

d) Put the registrar's name on the presentation and ask him in return to sign you off for procedures that you haven't managed to get done

e) Ask the registrar to review the presentation, make any required changes that evening, and present the amended presentation with his name on it the following day

Question 14: Suspecting a colleague of stealing

You are the house officer on a care of the elderly ward. The ward manager informs all members of the ward (clinical and non-clinical) that a number of medications including benzodiazepines and several packets of Co-codamol are unaccounted for in the medication cupboard. In the last couple of days, you have noticed one of your FY1 colleagues entering the treatment room, and emerging with what looks suspiciously like packets of medications stuffed inside his trouser pockets.

Rank in order the following actions in response to this situation *(1= Most appropriate; 5= Least appropriate)*

a) Keep your observations to yourself, as you do not wish to cause a fuss

b) Discretely ask the rest of the ward team if they've noticed anyone frequenting the treatment room more than usual

c) Utilise the camera on your phone to try and catch your colleague 'in the act'

d) Find your colleague and talk to him privately about your suspicions

e) Inform your consultant and ward manager that you suspect your colleague of stealing

Question 15: Providing medical advice to a colleague

Whilst on the ward a staff nurse with whom you enjoy a good relationship asks for your opinion about a sporting injury. A few days earlier she'd had an awkward fall whilst playing in a competitive hockey match. You have noticed that she has been having difficulty walking and looks to be in some discomfort.

Rank in order the following actions in response to this situation *(1= Most appropriate; 5= Least appropriate)*

a) Tell her that she will need to follow the PRICE* principle for what is likely to be a soft tissue injury

b) Tell her that you're concerned by her difficulty in walking and that she should go to the hospital's A&E department for an assessment

c) Find a quiet room on the ward to take a thorough history and examination before making a decision about what is to be done

d) Tell her she needs to inform her manager about the injury

e) Find an orthopaedic colleague and get him/her to see your nursing colleague to provide an expert opinion

*Protection Rest Ice Compression Elevation – conservative management for soft tissue injuries

Question 16: Prescribing practices

Whilst doing an evening ward cover shift, a nurse informs you that a medical patient needs intravenous (IV) fluids prescribed as he has not been eating or drinking well during the last couple of days. The fluids are due to run out at midnight and the nurse doesn't want to disturb the night doctor to prescribe the fluids. She informs you that the last set of IV fluids prescribed was a bag of 0.9% Normal Saline, running over 12 hours.

Rank in order the following actions in response to this situation *(1= Most appropriate; 5= Least appropriate)*

a) Review the patient's fluid balance chart and then prescribe fluids as appropriate

b) The patient will be asleep after midnight so wouldn't ordinarily be drinking any fluids, so tell the nurse that the patient won't need any fluids prescribed

c) Give a verbal order to prescribe 0.9% Normal Saline 1L over 12 hours

d) Assess the patient's hydration status clinically before prescribing any fluids

e) Encourage the patient to drink oral fluids so that he won't need any IV fluids

Question 17: Unwritten drug chart

It is 00.30 and you are at the end of a 13 hour on-call weekend shift in the Acute Admissions Department when you realise that you have forgotten to write the drug chart of one of the patients that you clerked that day. The patient is elderly and confused but not acutely unwell. The patient cannot provide a coherent history, but there is no one accompanying him and he does not have a list of his regular medications.

Rank in order the following actions in response to this situation *(1= Most appropriate; 5= Least appropriate)*

a) Hand the task over to the night team

b) Phone his next of kin to ask about his regular medication

c) Write up some PRN (as needed) basic analgesia and leave it for the day team to find out the regular medications

d) Look on the computer system for previous admissions and medications

e) Leave an entry in the notes for the day team/pharmacist to check with the GP the next morning

Question 18: Self-discharge

You are the medical house officer covering the night shift. You are looking after a 57 year old man who is on dialysis for end-stage renal failure. He was admitted to the medical ward with breathlessness and was successfully treated for pulmonary oedema and is now stable. You are called to see the gentleman as he now wants to self-discharge. He is due for his routine dialysis later this morning. When you arrive he looks well. However, as you review his blood test results you realise that his most recent potassium was 6.8mmol/L (normal 3.5-5.3mmol/L).

Rank in order the following actions in response to this situation (1= Most appropriate; 5= Least appropriate)

a) Offer him a 'discharge against medical advice' form and stress to him the importance of visiting his GP

b) Listen to the patient's concerns

c) Explain to the patient that a high potassium can cause dangerously abnormal heart rhythms

d) Call your senior colleague for advice

e) Obtain a repeat blood sample

Question 19: Sick leave

You are on a busy surgical ward round with one other FY1 and a consultant. Whilst on the ward round a nurse asks you to quickly write a sick leave form for a patient who is on his way to the discharge lounge following a laparoscopic appendicectomy. You are happy to write the form for ten days of sick leave. The nurse disagrees and insists the patient will need at least four weeks as she knows the patient's circumstances better.

Rank in order the following actions in response to this situation (1= Most appropriate; 5= Least appropriate)

a) Tell the nurse that you have no time to explore further than what you already know about the patient and if the sick leave needs to be extended, the patient can attend the GP surgery

b) Let the nurse know that sick leave authorisation is a doctor's decision

c) Tell the nurse you are still on the ward round and you will call the patient at home once discharged and post the sick leave form once the appropriate time has been decided by the team

d) Attend to the patient and complete the sick form accurately and return to the ward round as soon as possible, apologising to your team for your absence

e) Sign the form for four weeks as the nurse seems confident in her decision and return to ward round

Question 20: An angry pharmacist

Whilst in a discussion with a staff member, you are approached by a lady regarding one of your patients. She immediately launches into a verbal tirade about her mother's prescription chart. She states she is a qualified pharmacist and is appalled that her mother has been given Tramadol for pain relief when she expressly informed the admitting team that her mother tolerates it poorly. She states that her mother is now very confused and that no one on the ward knows anything about what the plan for her is. She says she will sue you and the hospital if her mother does not improve. You have only taken over the care of this patient earlier today.

Rank in order *the following actions in response to this situation (1= Most appropriate; 5= Least appropriate)*

a) Document the encounter in the patient's notes

b) Tell the patient's daughter that you will not speak to her unless she calms down

c) Ask the daughter to return to the patient's bedside and you will come and speak with her shortly after reviewing the notes

d) Review the drug chart and patient's notes to check whether or not any mention was made of an adverse reaction to Tramadol

e) Speak to your SHO about the situation

Question 21: You want my honest opinion?

A group of medical students have come for some clinical skills teaching as their final exams are a few months away. You happen to have a very pleasant patient who consents to being examined - a lower limb neurological examination. The student who examines the patient is nervous and only remembers to test light touch and proprioception; his examination technique is also poor. At the end of the session, the student brings his logbook for a signature under *'performed a peripheral neurological examination'*.

*Choose the **THREE most appropriate** actions to take in this situation*

a) Inform the student that you will sign on this occasion, however, he needs to improve, and thus should come back next week and perform the examination again

b) Advise the student that he might fail his finals if he doesn't revise his clinical skills and refuse to sign

c) Sign his logbook as a confidence building measure and comment that he 'wasn't too bad but can improve'

d) Ask him to come back later this week and perform the examination again for the signature

e) Encourage him to reflect on his examination and refuse to sign

f) Hold a democratic vote amongst the on-looking colleagues as to whether he deserves the signature

g) Sit with the student in a quiet room and ask him to talk you through the peripheral lower limb examination for the signature

h) Offer him material to read up on but don't sign

Question 22: Capacity versus confidentiality?

An elderly lady on the medical ward is being treated for an acute severe asthma attack; it is her second admission in three months. She has advanced Alzheimer's Disease and is deemed not to have mental capacity to make decisions on her health. Her daughter (next of kin) has come in to see her and you feel this would be an ideal opportunity to gain some information on possible environmental risk factors that may have precipitated the admissions. While the daughter temporarily leaves the ward to buy coffee, the patient asks you not to give her daughter any information about why she's in hospital.

*Choose the **THREE** most appropriate actions to take in this situation*

a) Arrange a convenient time to discuss the patient's condition with her daughter

b) Let the patient know she does not have mental capacity to make decisions and therefore the daughter needs to be informed

c) Accept the patient's wishes and do not disclose information to the daughter

d) Inform the nurses not to disclose any clinical information to the daughter

e) Kindly accept the patient's wishes but then go and discuss the case with her daughter

f) Apologetically reject the patient's wishes

g) Ask the daughter to speak to her mother and try to convince her to allow you to disclose information on her condition

h) Explain to the patient that you will need to disclose information and write your reasons for doing so in the notes

Question 23: A laxative mistake

There has been a mix up on the ward and it appears that the wrong patient was prescribed laxatives by one of the other doctors. Although no major medical consequences have occurred, the patient has had to take six trips to the toilet today and is understandably distressed by the mix up. You are the only doctor on the ward at the moment, and the patient approaches you very frustrated, accusing you of prescribing the laxatives, and demands you give your full name and GMC registration number.

*Choose the **THREE most appropriate** actions to take in this situation*

a) Explain to the patient that you did not prescribe the laxatives but will help find out who it was

b) Inform the patient you will only give him your GMC number if he calms down, despite not being the one who prescribed the medication

c) Threaten to call security if the patient doesn't calm down

d) Reluctantly give the patient your name and number whilst informing him of your innocence

e) Ignore the patient and leave the ward

f) Take the patient into a quiet room to explore his concerns

g) Ask a nurse, who witnessed the mix up, to vouch for your innocence in the hope of diffusing the situation

h) Refuse to hand your name and number over as you had nothing to do with the mix up

Question 24: Ditched by your SHO

You are an FY1 on a medical rotation. You realise that over the last few weeks, your SHO has been spending a lot of time in the office. He is either teaching medical students, or organising his CV and ePortfolio. His input towards the ward duties has been minimal. You are feeling increasingly stressed due to the increased workload. When you raise the issue with your SHO, he informs you that this is good experience for you and will help you in the long term. He also mentions that he had to do all of his F1 jobs himself with no help from his SHO and it helped him become a better doctor.

Choose the **THREE** *most appropriate actions to take in this situation*

a) Take on board the SHO's advice that this will be good for your training in the long-term

b) Speak to your registrar about the situation

c) Complain to your consultant about the situation

d) Disagree with your SHO and insist he shares the workload

e) Divide the workload with one of the final year medical students to enhance her experience and support her learning

f) Speak to the SHO on the other team about the situation

g) Instruct the nurses to bleep the SHO for any new ward jobs that arise

h) Do as many jobs as you can and leave the remaining jobs for the on-call doctor

Question 25: Challenging the SHO's decision?

You are in your first week of an elderly care medical rotation and you are reviewing the patients with your SHO on a junior ward round. You are asked to scribe the consultation of a lady known to have dementia who is awaiting a care home placement. The SHO is very brief with the patient and he does not explore her concerns in depth and does not formally examine the patient. At this point the SHO dictates for you to write: *'The patient is well and has no complaints. On examination, heart sounds normal and chest is clear and abdomen is soft and non-tender.'* You are aware that these findings have not been assessed formally, and the SHO senses your hesitation and reassures you that the consultant will review her tomorrow anyway.

*Choose the **THREE** most appropriate actions to take in this situation*

a) Ask the SHO to write his own notes as you are not happy to write this

b) Ask the SHO to examine the patient properly while still at the bed side

c) Inform the SHO that you will now be taking charge of the ward round in light of the patients' best interests

d) Tell your SHO that his conduct is unprofessional and request permission to leave the ward round

e) After the ward round, tell the SHO, clearly and assertively, that you refuse to document false information about patients

f) Inform your consultant about your SHO's behaviour

g) Apologise to the patient and explore her concerns

h) Write the statement and after you finish the ward round explore further why the SHO thinks it's ok to leave it for tomorrow

Question 26: Ward round prescribing

Whilst on a ward round reviewing patients post-operatively, you are asked to prescribe treatment for cellulitis for a patient who is four days post-op following a total abdominal hysterectomy and bilateral sapingo-oopherectomy. Your registrar asks you to prescribe Flucloxacillin as per guidelines (once every 6 hours). Later that day, the nurse rushes over to tell you that the patient's chest and abdomen are covered in a new red rash. When you look back at the drug chart you note that the allergy to Flucloxacillin is written at the front of the chart but not written inside the chart as is required in this trust.

*Choose the **THREE most appropriate** actions to take in this situation*

a) Advise the nurse to monitor the rash closely and if the patient's observations deteriorate, then to call you immediately

b) Call microbiology for advice on alternative therapy

c) Attend to the patient and ensure she is clinically stable

d) Explain to the patient why this error has occurred

e) Call your registrar and explain the error made on her ward round

f) Contact the dermatology consultant for an urgent review of the rash

g) Document the error as an incident form so this can be avoided in the future

h) Design an audit to analyse how well patients' allergy status are documented in your ward

Question 27: On call and unresponsive!

You have started a weekend on-call shift in your new medical rotation. You have a jobs list handed over to you and also carry an on-call ward bleep. You are reviewing a stable patient who had a fall on the ward. You receive another bleep about a patient who the nursing staff report needs to be assessed urgently as the patient seems unresponsive. The nurse is very abrupt and repeatedly says it's urgent and you should come to read the notes if you need more information. The nurse then asks you 'Are you coming now then or not?'.

*Choose the **THREE most appropriate** actions to take in this situation*

a) State that you will finish reviewing your current patient and then come to see the other patient straight away

b) Tell the nurse if she does not supply the relevant information you will not come to see the patient

c) Ask the nurse to use the SBAR* tool for the handover of information

d) Leave the patient you are reviewing and attend to the new patient

e) Ask her to put out a medical emergency call and start CPR

f) Tell the nurse that her request is very poorly communicated

g) Inform the nurse that you will bleep your registrar and inform him of the situation and act according to his advice

h) Inform your clinical supervisor and fill out an incident form

*SBAR – Situation/Background/Assessment/Recommendation

Question 28: The 'crash-call' relative

You are the first to arrive to a cardiac arrest call for a 35 year old female who is one day post-op following a pan-colectomy. With you are two staff nurses, and two FY1s. As you are ALS trained and the crash team is currently busy with another arrest call, you take command of the situation and lead the arrest. A short time into the arrest, the sister in charge informs you that the patient's husband has arrived and is asking whether he can observe the resuscitation. You are onto your fourth cycle of CPR and the prognosis is not good.

*Choose the **THREE most appropriate** actions to take in this situation*

a) Politely refuse the husband's request to observe the unfolding events

b) Ask the sister in charge to try and find local guidelines about relatives attending cardiac arrest calls

c) At the next rhythm check discuss with the members of the arrest team if they would mind the husband observing

d) Allow the husband to observe the arrest from a distance

e) Ask the sister in charge to explain to the husband that his wife is critical and that every attempt to resuscitate her is being made

f) Let the rest of the team continue with the arrest while you speak to the husband

g) Inform the sister in charge that you'd like to have a thorough discussion with the husband later

h) Explain to the husband through the curtain that the prognosis is not good and that the team need to concentrate on providing the best care to his wife

Question 29: Prioritising your workload

You're working on a surgical firm when a fellow FY1 who is on-call for the surgical teams asks you to hold his bleep for 30 minutes so he can get some lunch without being disturbed as he is quite tired. He tells you that there are only two non-urgent jobs and that if there are any problems, to contact the registrar on-call. You agree to help out, having first-hand experience of being on-call only last week, you remember the difficulty you had in getting lunch. Unfortunately, the on-call bleep goes off after a couple of minutes, and it's the registrar asking for you to assist her in theatre, immediately.

*Choose the **THREE most appropriate** actions to take in this situation*

a) Inform the on-call registrar that you are just covering for your colleague whilst he gets lunch and that you cannot assist her in theatre at the moment

b) Inform your team that you are needed in theatre

c) Find another FY1 to cover you while you go to theatre to assist

d) Inform your FY1 colleague who is on-call that he's needed in theatre immediately

e) Consult your jobs list and delegate any jobs that are urgent

f) Tell your on-call FY1 colleague that he's needed in theatre and to take over from you once he has finished lunch

g) Rush to theatre immediately

h) Clarify with the on-call registrar the type of surgery and expected duration before making a decision to assist or not

Question 30: The battle for annual leave

You want to book annual leave for a long overdue trip to the USA. You've arranged an informal swap for an on-call medical weekend with a fellow FY1 so that you can have two weeks holiday. The week before you're due to fly out, your FY1 colleague informs you that due to unforeseen circumstances, he is unable to work the weekend you've swapped. There is no one else on the rota you can swap with as it's close to change over time for all the FY1s.

*Choose the **THREE most appropriate** actions to take in this situation*

a) Ask the rota coordinator whether she can arrange a locum doctor to work the weekend in question

b) Inform your colleague that it's his responsibility to find someone to work the weekend that you'd agreed to swap

c) Claim that you're sick during the weekend you're meant to be on-call so that you can go on holiday

d) Try and find a FY1 from another specialty to work your weekend and work a weekend of his/her choice in return

e) Amend your holiday plans, so that you return in time to work your weekend on-call

f) Ask a friend who is an FY1 at another hospital trust to work your on-call weekend

g) Arrange a meeting with the leave coordinator and the FY1 with whom you had swapped the shift

h) As you've already swapped the shift and your plans are set, ignore your fellow FY1s problem of not being able to work your original weekend

Practice Paper
1
Answers

Question 1: Home time!

This scenario is based upon the GMC guideline that states:

'In providing care you must:

(a) prescribe drugs or treatment, including repeat prescriptions, only when you have adequate knowledge of the patient's health and are satisfied that the drugs or treatment serve the patient's needs.' (Good Medical Practice, paragraph 16a).

The correct ranking of options in this scenario are:

B.D.C.E.A.

B - Inform the nurse your shift has finished but offer the bleep number for the next doctor on shift

Following this guideline, it is important to keep in mind that unless you are willing to assess the patient, you should not prescribe any medication, particularly Ibuprofen, which has potentially serious adverse effects such as gastrointestinal bleeding, renal failure and bronchoconstriction to patients who are susceptible. It is unfair for you to have to stay behind longer than you already have, particularly as the patient is not acutely unwell and additionally because you may be tired. However, it would be in the best interest of the patient for you to offer the nurse the bleep number of the doctor on shift as this would also show initiative. If you were not overcome with tiredness, it would be supportive to look through the patient's notes and review the patient at the bedside for any contraindications to the drug, bearing in mind that the patient is in pain - however you are under no obligation to do this.

D - Refuse to sign and inform her that the other doctor knows the patient better

All the following options fail to use initiative or offer a reasonable course of action for the nurse to take. However, option D is in keeping with the guidelines and provides a perfectly fair justification to the nurse as to why you cannot sign the chart.

C - Ignore the nurse's request and tell her your shift has finished

The following three answers are all very poor courses of action to take. Whilst it may seem unfair to 'ignore the nurse', it is an even unhealthier approach to encourage the nurse to file a complaint (option E) in such a situation. This is because the doctor may have had to attend to other more urgent matters and therefore could have a legitimate reason for being late.

E - Return the pen torch, advise the nurse to file a complaint against the doctor, then leave

This is similar to the option above in that it is saying, in so many words, to also ignore the nurse. However, the additional information you are giving the nurse here is not that your shift has finished, but rather to file a complaint, which is uncalled for in these circumstances.

A - Sign the drug chart and thank the nurse for the pen torch

In keeping with the guideline and the explanation for option B, this is the least appropriate course of action to take of the options given as it is an unsafe approach to adopt.

Question 2: Hospital or hotel?

This scenario draws guidance from the following statement within the GMC Good Medical Practice:

'You must not refuse or delay treatment because you believe that a patient's actions or lifestyle have contributed to their condition.' (Good Medical Practice, paragraph 57).

The correct ranking for this question is:

D.A.E.B.C.

D - Ask him to sit on his chair, prescribe him his Chlordiazepoxide and ask the nurse to bring his lunch

While it appears that this patient is insensitive to the continuous admissions over the past month, this does not negate the fact that he should still be treated. It appears that the discharge plan has not been comprehensive enough and so indicates that further thought needs to be put into it to avoid regular admissions. As there are immediate medical needs of the patient that require addressing, he should be appropriately treated as soon as possible. This should, in turn, help to calm him down.

A - Explain to him that if he continues to misbehave you will have to call security

The remaining options deal more with his behaviour than his current health. Option A may help to calm him down for the time being and thus addresses the more immediate needs of the situation, and of the safety of the surrounding patients.

E - Discuss the situation with social services

Social services have a dedicated team who can help address complex discharge issues. While this case may require support from security initially, due to the patient's behaviour, it would be important to involve social services to deal with the longer term needs of this patient. Option A has been preferred as it prioritises the more immediate needs first.

B - Inform him that he needs to sign up for an alcohol support service to improve his behaviour

While this is a reasonable option, it has no bearing on the immediate scenario, particularly considering the patient has refused the offer of support groups in the past.

C - Ignore him for the time being as this should act as behavioural conditioning for his demeanour and repetitive admissions

The patient is medically unwell due to the alcohol withdrawal and so in following the GMC guidelines, should not be refused care.

Question 3: Cremation Form

This scenario considers the circumstances when one's personal beliefs may conflict with clinical practice. It is advisable to be aware of such situations and to read the Good Medical Practice (paragraph 54) as well as the related Personal Beliefs and Medical Practice guidelines to understand the appropriate steps to take. In relation to this scenario, the following guidelines encompass what is being tested:

'You must be considerate to those close to the patient, and be sensitive and responsive in giving them information and support.' (Good Medical Practice, paragraph 33).

'You must not express your personal beliefs (including political, religious and moral beliefs) to patients in ways that exploit their vulnerability or are likely to cause them distress.' (Good Medical Practice, paragraph 54).

The correct ranking for this question is therefore:

C.A.B.E.D.

C - Ask one of your medical colleagues who has seen the body to sign the form instead

Rather than raise your objections to cremation in the midst of a sensitive event, it would be most appropriate to ask a colleague to sign the form in order for the process to occur swiftly and efficiently for the grieving family. For a colleague to be able to sign the form they are required to have been involved in the care of the patient within the current hospital admission.

A - Apologise and explain to the family member that you will be unable to sign the form but another colleague can

Of the remaining options, it is appropriate to show honesty and integrity in informing the family of your personal beliefs, while at the same time reassuring them that a colleague will be able to sign the form.

B - Sign the form reluctantly

This is not an ideal option for you to take, and usually there would be another colleague who can sign the form. However, in relation to the scenario and remaining options, it would be most appropriate for you to sign and not to delay the signature further. Furthermore, in analysing the language of the scenario, you are claimed to 'prefer' not to sign as opposed to, for example, being adamant, and thus hints at a slight sense of willingness on your part were you required to sign. This option is preferred to option E as it would be unreasonable for you to 'arrange a date' to discuss the situation. This would prolong the anxiety of the grieving family, whose emotions should be put ahead of yours in such circumstances.

E - Arrange a date to discuss the situation with your clinical supervisor

Arranging a meeting with your clinical supervisor would not address the needs of this sensitive situation, but this option would nevertheless be favoured above the following answer that could cause more harm than good and breaks fundamental GMC guidelines.

D - Offer alternative avenues the family may wish to explore other than cremating the body

Whilst you may have an objection to a certain practice, this does not deem it appropriate to use the opportunity to dissuade a patient or family from their desired decision. This would be an insensitive approach to take in the current circumstances and could warrant a complaint from an emotional family member. The following GMC statement outlines the guidelines on such an approach:

'You must not impose your beliefs on patients, or cause distress by the inappropriate or insensitive expression of religious, political or other beliefs or views. Equally, you must not put pressure on patients to discuss or justify their beliefs (or the absence of them).' (Personal Beliefs and Medical Practice Guidelines, paragraph 19).

Question 4: Yellow card, surely?

This scenario aims to test one's ability to prioritise tasks, and includes a learning point on reporting adverse drug reactions.

The correct answers for this question are:

A.D.E.B.C.

A - Sit with her and listen to her concerns and fears

The most important action is to console the patient, especially as she is emotionally distressed. It usually only takes a few minutes and it goes a long way in improving the patient's mental well being.

D - Send a report to the Medicines and Healthcare products Regulatory Agency and let her know how to do the same

The GMC guidelines state:

'When prescribing for a patient you should:

(c) inform the Medicines and Healthcare products Regulatory Agency of adverse reactions to medicines reported by your patients in accordance with the Yellow Card Scheme. You should provide patients with information about how to report suspected adverse reactions through the patient Yellow Card Scheme.' (Good Practice in Prescribing Medicines, paragraph 6c).

The Yellow Card Scheme encourages both doctors and patients to report adverse drug reactions via their website, helping to regulate the safety of drugs being prescribed. Although they welcome reports of any drug or reaction, they state that they are particularly interested in reactions that have not been accounted for within the drug information sheet or those which interfere with a patient's life. Within this scenario, the drug reaction was said to be 'severe and rare', indicating that not much was known about the side effect and it had adverse effects on the patient.

E - Take a minute out to call your friends and say that you'll be late for the planned football match tonight

This option demonstrates your willingness to re-arrange plans as a direct result of patient care and shows compliance with GMC guidance of placing the patient as the first concern. Doctors may have social commitments that can occasionally interfere with work, and it is important to stay in control and avoid mismanagement of one's time. In this scenario taking 'a few minutes' out to organise your social plans will efficiently help to limit any stress and pressure you may feel to leave on time, and allows further focus on your patient(s).

B - Ask the ward pharmacist to give you an overview on drug reactions

While this option is certainly beneficial and shows initiative, it does not show immediate concern for the patient, particularly when considering it as a stand-alone option in relation to the scenario. When compared relative to the other options, answers A and D are important for patient safety, whilst option E is also indirectly relevant to patients by freeing up your out-of-work commitments. Furthermore, pharmacists also have tasks of their own and may not always be readily available for teaching.

C - File a complaint against the doctor who prescribed the penicillin

This option is unnecessary and incorrect as the doctor was not in the wrong. The patient was not known to have any drug allergies and therefore this option will act negatively upon team relations.

Question 5: Medical students arrive for teaching

Teaching students is essential for passing on knowledge and skills to the next generation of doctors. Students can learn via direct teaching or opportunistic learning within a clinical setting. Teaching also helps to consolidate your own knowledge; as the mantra goes 'see one, do one, teach one'. It is thus essential to help train prospective doctors to the best of your ability. The GMC provide guidelines on teaching, outlined in the following paragraph:

'You should be prepared to contribute to teaching and training doctors and students.' (Good Medical Practice, paragraph 39).

B.D.E.C.A.

B - Ask the students to write down the steps of venepuncture as a group, whilst you collect the equipment, and then to observe you

Doctors are often busy, and so cannot let that dictate whether or not they will be able to teach. One should be prepared to be opportunistic and provide teaching without compromising patient care. Students learn in different ways and the objective of being within a clinical setting is to understand how medical theory is put into practice. It is always beneficial to observe a practical procedure before attempting one, particularly in this scenario. For fresh third year students this would be the optimal option. Further, rather than asking the students to simply observe (option D), it would be best to promote learning using different methods, while at the same time not affecting your busy task list.

D - Ask the students to accompany you on your jobs and to just observe

As above, observation is a vital step in learning, especially when performing practical tasks, and so one should not feel they are doing an injustice to the students' learning opportunities by offering this.

E - Refer the students over to the doctors' mess to find a colleague who is free and can teach them

Whilst a doctor with free time will be able to go round to wards and find good patients for the students to examine, the option does not guarantee that the students will find a suitable and willing doctor to teach them at the mess, and therefore may be a hindrance to their learning.

C - Go with them and supervise each one as they attempt to take blood

Not only will this be a hasty step to take for students who are at the beginning of their clinical career ('first day'), it will also delay the tasks at hand and potentially compromise patient care. It is also stated that there are a 'group' of students, and therefore to supervise each would further delay jobs. It would therefore be preferable, in this scenario, to choose option E above C for the sake of patient safety over student learning. However, both are inappropriate steps to take.

A - Give a brief overview of venepuncture, delegate the students a patient each, and tell them to report back to you once they're done taking blood

This is a dangerous approach to take and can compromise patient care. You will be responsible for any problems that may arise. With regards to this option, it is important to consider the GMC guidance:

'You must make sure that all staff you manage have appropriate supervision.' (Good Medical Practice, paragraph 40).

Question 6: Nobody has to know?

Regardless of the cause of death, confidentiality of the deceased patient should be respected. Although there are conditions where disclosure may be appropriate, as outlined within the GMC Confidentiality guidelines, the general principle is as follows:

'Your duty of confidentiality continues after a patient has died...If the patient had asked for information to remain confidential, you should usually respect their wishes.' (GMC Confidentiality, paragraph 70).

This indicates the following order to be most appropriate:

C.A.E.D.B.

C - Inform him that it is too early to be sure and a post-mortem may be required, but you will inform a senior to sit down and speak to him soon

This approach is honest and errs on the side of caution. It protects you from saying anything untrue at this point without foreknowledge. Furthermore, this situation is quite complex, and so when discussing the cause of death it may be appropriate for a senior colleague with more experience to sit down with the family. This option maintains confidentiality.

A - Inform him that the exact cause of death isn't clear and this condition can occur spontaneously which may be the case with his wife

Although option A is being partially dishonest, it may be seen as the lesser of two wrongs as disclosure of the cause of death would be going against the wife's requests. This said, pulmonary embolisms can occur spontaneously and there are other risk factors that predispose to the condition. Therefore, this approach is not completely dishonest and the option is relatively, a more appropriate choice to make than those below.

E - Explain to him that you have a suspicion, however, you can't be sure until you have discussed it with your seniors

The following options are not ideal, however, they must be assessed relative to one another. Whilst option E will give the husband an unwarranted sense of expectation that you will disclose your 'suspicion', and therefore cause potential problems, it delays any potential disclosure until the discussion with a senior takes place and thus maintains patient confidentiality for the time being at least.

D - Take a brief sexual history from him and ascertain from his knowledge whether there was a chance that Mrs Liston could have been pregnant

This is completely inappropriate and hints at the possible cause of death. However, it does not completely disclose the cause and therefore relative to option .B, is a less severe breach of confidentiality.

B - Take him into a quiet room and explain to him honestly that her pregnancy may have been the underlying reason for her death

This option contravenes GMC guidelines with regards to respecting confidentiality of patients who have passed away. Furthermore, this could cause unforeseen problems within the family had the wife become pregnant by someone else, especially considering her request that 'nobody has to know'.

Question 7: An ideal catch – I think I've found 'the one'

Trust is a key component of the doctor-patient relationship and the most effective way of securing this trust is by maintaining professional boundaries at all times. One should not allow emotional relationships to interfere with his/her care of a patient, thereby obscuring objective decision-making and management. The GMC guidelines state:

'In order to maintain professional boundaries, and the trust of patients and the public, you must not establish or pursue a sexual or improper emotional relationship with a patient.' (Maintaining Boundaries, paragraph 4).

To this end, the most appropriate order is:

D.C.E.B.A.

D - Decline the offer and inform a senior that you no longer feel comfortable with her behaviour and suggest whether it would be better to hand the patient over to the team on the other half of the ward

This may seem drastic, however, it is superior to all the other options in this scenario. Primarily, it coincides with GMC guidelines of not pursuing improper emotional relationships with patients, and it also takes into consideration that your clinical judgement was affected by this patient's remarks by almost forgetting to take bloods from her. This indicates that it would be sensible and safe to hand her over to the care of other colleagues in order to help prevent any potential clinical mishaps from occurring.

C - Explain to Miss Parker that her comments have been completely inappropriate and that you have no interest in dating anyone right now, then leave and take a minute to think about the situation

Whilst this may come across as harsh, it is the most appropriate action to take relative to the remaining options. Options B and A are in contradiction to GMC guidelines, and only option E can be compared to C. However, option E does not deal with the issue at hand and may instead encourage her further. This could once again impair your clinical performance and potentially be harmful to the patient. Option C shows that you have attempted to explain the situation to her and reflect on what should be done, as opposed to letting it pass.

E - Smile at Miss Parker and crack a joke, then carry on with your jobs on the ward

As explained above.

B - Inform Miss Parker that your primary aim is to get her feeling better and out of hospital, after this is achieved you can discuss the matter further

This appears reasonable on first glance, but it contravenes the GMC guidance above, as it encourages the behaviour from the patient, and it further contravenes supplementary GMC guidance as outlined below:

'Pursuing a sexual relationship with a former patient may be inappropriate, regardless of the length of time elapsed since the therapeutic relationship ended. This is because it may be difficult to be certain that the professional relationship is not being abused.' (Maintaining Boundaries, paragraph 6).

A - Inform Miss Parker that you need time to think about it, however, you might be interested in her offer

This is in contradiction with the GMC principle of not establishing improper emotional relationships with patients, in particular one in which your clinical judgement is being affected.

Question 8: Up to mischief

This scenario deals with probity, and the importance of being honest and open when faced with matters such as criminal convictions. Doctors must uphold the trust given to them within their profession, and ensure that their conduct outside of work is in agreement with the law. If a doctor's actions break national or international law, it is their duty to inform the GMC of this, as summarised:

'You must tell us without delay if, anywhere in the world:

a you have accepted a caution from the police or been criticised by an official inquiry

b you have been charged with or found guilty of criminal offence

c another professional body has made a finding against your registration as a result of fitness to practise procedures.' (Good Medical Practice, paragraph 75).

B.C.E.A.D.

B - Phone up the GMC and tell them what just happened as well as last month's incident

The GMC have a short supplementary guidance on 'Reporting criminal and regulatory proceedings within and outside the UK' where offences are discussed in line with the principle above, including driving fines, Anti-Social Behaviour Orders (ASBO) and possession of illegal drugs, amongst other convictions. On receiving a warning for the possession of cannabis, the GMC must be informed:

'The use or possession of illegal drugs may raise a question about a doctor's fitness to practise, so you must also tell the GMC if you receive a warning for the possession of cannabis.'

(Reporting criminal and regulatory proceedings within and outside the UK, paragraph 8).

In keeping with probity and honesty it would also be relevant to inform the GMC of the incident last month, more so if you were given an ASBO.

C - Seek advice from your defence body in case it affects your GMC registration

The next most appropriate course of action to take is informing a defence body of the situation who can advise you on the best course of action to take:

'If you are unsure whether or not to inform the GMC about any of the matters...you should seek advice from a defence body, medical association or from the GMC.' (Reporting criminal and regulatory proceedings within and outside the UK, paragraph 10).

E - Carry out an internet search just to make sure this doesn't affect your medical profession

In reality, were you not to be sure this would certainly be a very reasonable approach to take. However, on knowledge of the guidelines, this is not the most appropriate course of action to take and the above options are relatively more correct.

A - Count your lucky stars and stay on your best behaviour for the rest of the trip

This option contravenes the guidelines and is therefore not advisable. It lacks the probity and honesty required of a GMC registered doctor.

D - Turn over a new leaf and sell the rest of the cannabis you had saved in the flat

This is a criminal offence and could result in up to 14 years in prison or a fine, or both, according to current UK drug laws.

Question 9: A case of child abuse

The guidelines on this issue are clear:

'Whether or not you have vulnerable adults or children and young people as patients, you should consider their needs and welfare and offer them help if you think their rights have been abused or denied.'

(Good Medical Practice, paragraph 27).

Every trust and place of work will have very clear policies on how to manage situations when you have concerns about the welfare of a child.

D.B.C.E.A.

D - Discuss the case with your seniors/senior nursing staff

Your first action should be to discuss the case with another senior member of staff. This may be the ward sister, senior doctor or the assigned safeguarding children officer. They will have detailed knowledge of the appropriate steps to take and will help guide your actions

B - Call the social services team

If option D is not possible (e.g. out of hours) then contacting the duty social worker would be the next appropriate step. Your senior may also suggest this as the next appropriate management step.

C - Call the police

Calling the police should only be done where there is immediate danger to the child.

E - Get a collateral history from the girl's father

Getting a collateral history from the father may have some use but should be undertaken by the appropriate members of the social services team. In the immediate instance this may also put the child in danger.

A - Try to convince her to let you get help for her but assure her you will not tell anyone if she does not want you to

The Children Act 1989 permits the sharing of information to safeguard children where failure to do so may expose a child to risk of serious harm. So although the co-operation of the child should be sought, it is not essential.

If you are in any doubt the answer is always option D – discuss with your seniors.

Question 10: Family pressure

The correct order for this scenario is:

A.D.E.C.B.

'You must listen to patients, take account of their views, and respond honestly to their questions.'

(Good Medical Practice, paragraph 31).

A - Ask the patient if she has expressed these thoughts to anyone else and explore her feelings further

The most appropriate immediate action would be to explore the patient's views. This will allow you to gain a better insight into the patient's concerns and take a more individualised approach to her ongoing care.

D - Empathise with her thoughts and explain you will inform your consultant

Active listening and acting upon the patient's concerns will not only be in the patient's best interests, but will also act to improve the doctor-patient relationship. The ultimate decision on whether she has the operation or not will be made by the patient when she discusses the matter with the consultant, therefore, it would be relevant and necessary for you to refer her concerns on to your senior team member.

E - Tell the patient you will ask one of the specialist cancer nurses to come and talk to her about these concerns

Although specialist nurses are often well placed to explore these issues with patients, there is no reason why you should not initially act to build the doctor-patient relationship by exploring her concerns. The two previous options involve exploring the patient's worries further before referring her elsewhere.

C - Tell her you will cancel her operation and you can refer her to the MacMillan nursing team

You do not have the expertise, and neither is it your responsibility to advise the patient that their operation should be cancelled and a change of management strategy instigated.

B - Tell her not to worry, the team will look after her and things will be ok

To ignore and dismiss the patient's concerns goes against the clear GMC guidance given above. Furthermore, it is not advisable to tell the patient that everything is going to be okay even if you are trying to console her, as there is a chance that this may not be the case and things may not be okay.

Question 11: A flexible what?

The correct order for this scenario is:

C.D.E.A.B.

C - Speak to your registrar about your concerns over the patient's understanding of what was said

Discussing your concerns with the registrar must be a priority here. It is a busy post-take round, and it is possible that in a bid to see all the patients quickly, important details have been missed, such as ensuring full and proper consent for an invasive procedure has been obtained. In discussing this with your registrar, you will display professionalism and trustworthiness in your efforts to do what is best for the patient.

D - Speak to the nurse in charge and request a translator for the patient

For patients who do not speak English as a first language, it is important to properly assess whether they are able to consent to a procedure and fully understand the implications of accepting/refusing to have it. As stated in the GMC's guidelines:

'You must be satisfied that you have consent or other valid authority before you carry out any examination or investigation, provide treatment or involve patients or volunteers in teaching or research.' (Good Medical Practice, paragraph 17).

Further advice is outlined in the 'New Doctor' guidelines, paragraph 9, that junior doctors must *'d) demonstrate that they encourage and support effective communication with people, both individually and in groups, including people with learning disabilities and those who do not have English as their main language.'*

Another important aspect of this scenario is patient trust in the medical team. If this patient were to undergo a flexible sigmoidoscopy without fully appreciating what it entails, she may lose trust in health professionals for subjecting her to a procedure without ensuring she understood what it was, and without being offered the opportunity to accept/refuse it.

E - Fill out the request form but hold on to it until you feel the patient fully understands the proposed procedure

This is a logical step that follows C and D. Filling out request forms after seeing patients saves time and often patient details are best filled out having just seen the patient where their clinical history is fresh in your mind. This form can then be taken down as soon as consent is obtained, or correctly disposed off if refused. Full documentation of the consent process should be made in the patient's notes.

A - Drop the form off to endoscopy and try to re-consent the patient after the round

This would not be acceptable as the patient has not consented and should therefore, not be put on an endoscopy list. She could conceivably take up the slot of a patient who has consented and it is very possible that she may go down for her procedure before you have a chance to get back to her after a busy round. There is also a real risk of subjecting the patient to harm if she is unable to follow instructions during the procedure because of the language barrier. You are not in a position in this scenario to consent a patient as you have not been delegated to do so by the registrar, thereby undermining his authority and going against GMC guidelines:

'If you are the doctor undertaking an investigation or providing treatment, it is your responsibility to discuss it with the patient. If this is not practical, you can delegate the responsibility to someone else, provided you make sure that the person you delegate to:

> a) *Is suitably trained and qualified*
> b) *Has sufficient knowledge of the proposed investigation or treatment, and understands the risks involved*
> c) *Understands, and agrees to act in accordance with, the guidance in this booklet.'*

(GMC Consent: patients and doctors making decisions together, paragraph 26).

B - Drop the form off to endoscopy without trying to re-consent as this procedure is being done in the patient's best interests

This is the most inappropriate course of action. The patient was not able to consent to the procedure and as such, no attempts should be made to request the procedure until proper consent is obtained. Although option A goes against guidelines, it makes an attempt at keeping patient safety at the forefront, which is the overriding principle in all cases.

Question 12: Feedback to the boss!

Feedback often feels like an extra job that can be de-prioritised at work, and the benefits of constructive feedback are not always appreciated. Therefore one may have a tendency to feel apathetic towards delivering feedback and feel it may be easier to write what is simple and favourable for the individual receiving the feedback. However, the GMC outlines this as unacceptable for any doctor:

'You must be honest and objective when writing references, and when appraising or assessing the performance of colleagues, including locums and students. References must include all information relevant to your colleagues' competence, performance and conduct.' (Good Medical Practice, paragraph 41).

Based on this, the answers are ordered as follows:

C.A.B.D.E.

C - Complete the feedback form accurately describing all the areas of concern you have where appropriate, even if you know this may count badly against you in future forms and references

Fear of providing bad feedback is a concern for many but is usually baseless and rarely comes to be a problem. In any case, it should not deter you from your primary role to provide honest and accurate comments. It should, however, be an area that you flag up to your educational supervisor at an early stage and they will usually talk to you about your concerns. While you are the only junior doctor on the team, the nature of feedback forms ensures confidentiality is maintained. It would be highly unlikely that comments are traced back to you.

A - Appreciate that you are a junior and therefore try to make your comments inoffensive and toned down, while still attempting to convey most of your views across

It is important to remember your role and that inoffensive feedback is always recommended. Nevertheless, the nature of this appraisal is one that acknowledges your role as a junior doctor and therefore honest, accurate, informative and constructive comments are fundamental and should be how feedback is given. A doctor should not feel the need to restrict their feedback, particularly when considering the practise of the consultant described within the scenario.

B - Avoid completing the feedback form in case it will affect your working relationship and discuss your concerns with your educational supervisor instead

If you have serious concern that the feedback may have a negative effect to your future career, then you should discuss the matter with your educational supervisor before completing the form. This is not the most preferable course of action as it avoids giving beneficial feedback, however, at the same time, it involves seeking advice from a suitable senior.

D - Before completing the form, discuss your concerns with other colleagues in the mess to ensure that this is not only your view and/or a misunderstanding

It is not recommended to discuss feedback informally amongst colleagues within or outside your team. Feedback should remain confidential where appropriate and if you feel discussion with others is needed, then this should be done in a professional setting and manner.

E - Complete the form in a positive way that will hopefully reflect in your own feedback from the consultant

In no scenario should a doctor give feedback inaccurately. This feedback system is part of the indirect system to improve patient care and is in all patients' best interest. This option is therefore inappropriate.

Question 13: I want my name on the audit

This scenario assesses the junior doctor's commitment to professionalism and ability to work effectively as a part of a team.
This may appear to be an easy situation in theory but it is difficult in practice. People should only be credited for work they have done, to do otherwise is to be disingenuous, unprofessional and will ultimately lead to patient safety issues when unqualified individuals are put in positions of responsibility based on work they haven't done. This said, as a junior you may feel obliged to help your senior. Ultimately, professionalism in the guise of honesty and integrity are the most important factors.

E.B.A.C.D.

E - Ask the registrar to review the presentation, make any required changes that evening, and present the amended presentation with his name on it the following day

This is the ideal outcome as it reconciles both of the potentially conflicting principles stated above. The senior doctor is able to review the presentation and potentially improve it. Allowing him to present the audit gives him enough credit to warrant his name on the research. Such honesty is emphasised by the GMC:

'You must act with honesty and integrity when designing, organising, or carrying out research, and follow national research governance guidelines and our guidance.'

(Good Medical Practice, paragraph 67).

B - Decline but offer to help him on another joint audit

This is the next best option as it maintains the professional integrity of the trainee, but also offers a solution to a potentially awkward situation. It is hard for a junior not to follow a direct request from a senior, however, such probity should be understood and respected by all colleagues.

A - Decline, as the registrar has not made a contribution to the work so it would be unethical

This is technically correct but it does not offer a solution and may lead to a strained working relationship and as such, is less preferable to options E or B.

C - Put the registrar's name on the presentation

This is possibly the easiest choice to make in the immediate setting. However, it is unethical and inappropriate and if allowed to happen, such unprofessional behaviour could ultimately lead to issues affecting patient safety and put into question both the registrar's and your own probity.

D - Put the registrar's name on the presentation and ask him in return to sign you off for procedures that you haven't managed to get done

This is the least favourable option as it demonstrates dishonest behaviour that, as explained above, can also lead to poor patient care. Here, the junior doctor is actively complicit in the deceitful behaviour.

Question 14: Suspecting a colleague of stealing

Key themes this question tests are from 'The duties of a doctor registered with the General Medical Council', found on the first page of the Good Medical Practice guidelines:

'Take prompt action if you think that patient safety, dignity or comfort is being compromised.'

'Be honest and open and act with integrity.'

'Never discriminate unfairly against patients or colleagues.'

The correct order for this scenario is:

D.E.B.C.A.

D - Find your colleague and talk to him privately about your suspicions

You have no evidence of any wrong-doing, just a suspicion. It is best to discuss your concerns directly with your colleague to clear up any doubt and hopefully establish some facts.

E - Inform your consultant and ward manager that you suspect your colleague of stealing

It would be advisable to first clarify any suspicions with the colleague in question, and then if doubt still remains, you do not need to wait for conclusive evidence of misconduct and should escalate matters to the consultant on your team, as outlined in the following guidelines:

'Wherever possible, you should first raise your concern with your manager or an appropriate officer of the organisation you have a contract with or which employs you – such as the consultant in charge of the team...' (GMC Raising and acting on concerns about patient safety, paragraph 13).

'You do not need to wait for proof - you will be able to justify raising a concern if you do so honestly, on the basis of reasonable belief and through appropriate channels, even if you are mistaken.' (GMC Raising and acting on concerns about patient safety, paragraph 10c).

B - Discretely ask the rest of the ward team if they've noticed anyone frequenting the treatment room more than usual

This is a mediocre response to the situation, as it does not directly aim to deal with the situation as the preceding two ptions, but at the same time does not cause any harm or neglect. It may be argued that this option could help to confirm your suspicions. However, whether or not there is a consensus that your colleague has been entering the treatment room regularly does not provide any further evidence of stealing. Therefore, along with the GMC guidance above, it would be best to escalate concerns as soon as possible based on current observations.

C - Utilise the camera on your phone to try and catch your colleague 'in the act'

One cannot condone spying on their colleague. However in this scenario, it is relatively more appropriate than option A as it shows an attempt to rectify the situation. In not doing anything (option A), there is a potential for patient care to be affected due to the lack of medications and also neglects the potential misconduct and well being of your colleague, which could also have an indirect effect on patient care.

A - Keep your observations to yourself, as you do not wish to cause a fuss

Doing nothing doesn't solve the fundamental problem of the theft of medication; it also belies the fact that you may have a colleague who is in need of help (and thus may be compromising their ability to be an effective doctor). It further calls into question your own probity.

Question 15: Providing medical advice to a colleague

This is a common occurrence, as a doctor, other members of staff as well friends and family will seek ad-hoc medical advice from you. This scenario relates to The GMC's Good Medical Practice: Avoiding treating those close to you (paragraph 16g):

'wherever possible, avoid providing medical care to yourself or anyone with whom you have a close personal relationship'.

The correct order for this scenario is thus:

D.B.C.E.A.

D - Tell her she needs to inform her manager about the injury

There are hospital policies regarding illness and injuries. This nurse's injury may be significant enough to require medical attention and may also be impairing her ability to work. She should seek advice from her manager in the first instance - thus allowing cover for her duties if it was deemed that she was not fit enough to continue working at the present time.

B - Tell her that you're concerned by her difficulty in walking and that she should go to the hospital's A&E department for an assessment

It is safer for the nurse to be assessed formally in an area where investigations and tests can be carried out such as in the A&E department, and where a formal history and examination can be taken.

C - Find a quiet room on the ward to take a thorough history and examination before making a decision about what is to be done

This is not recommended. There should be continuity of care after such a consultation and so it is best to follow a formal route of investigation as explained above. This is better than referring to an orthopaedic colleague, however, as you would be able to perform basic initial assessments before jumping to a decision of involving a specialist.

E - Find an orthopaedic colleague and get him/her to see your nursing colleague to provide an expert opinion

This option is not ideal even if it is a specialist's opinion as the assessment is not being done in a formal setting, and thus there will be restrictions on further investigations/management as well as the lack of continuity of care.

A - Tell her that she will need to follow the PRICE* principle for what is likely to be a soft tissue injury

This advice is poor, as you have no idea of the extent of the injury and the consequence of this could be serious should this nurse have, for example, a fractured foot/ankle.

Literature from the medical insurance/defence unions states that by providing medical advice you should either ensure the patient has appropriate follow up (GP, specialist etc.) or you must follow up yourself. If you are to provide advice, you should take a clear history and examine the appropriate system, and make clear documentations. In all instances you should advise your colleague/friend/relative that they should seek formal medical advice.

Question 16: Prescribing practices

The correct ranking of options for this scenario is:

D.A.E.B.C.

D - Assess the patient's hydration status clinically before prescribing any fluids

This answer adopts the most common sense approach as the patient's current hydration status is the most important sign indicating whether or not the patient requires fluids. As with any medication you prescribe, IV fluids can only be administered if there is a clinical indication. This would involve looking through the patient's notes, observation chart, fluid-balance chart, blood results, taking a brief history from the patient and clinically examining their needs.

A - Review the patient's fluid balance chart and then prescribe fluids as appropriate

An objective analysis of a patient's fluid balance chart will help form your judgement as to whether a patient needs fluid or not. However, this should be used in conjunction with the patient's clinical signs to determine their fluid requirements.

E - Encourage the patient to drink oral fluids so that he won't need any IV fluids

If the patient is well enough and there are no contraindications, it may be reasonable to encourage the patient to drink oral fluids. However, this is not the number one choice here as we have been told that the patient has been on IV fluids due to poor oral intake. This is more appropriate than B as it at least makes an attempt to encourage fluid intake.

B - The patient will be asleep after midnight so wouldn't ordinarily be drinking any fluids, so tell the nurse that the patient won't need any fluids prescribed

While the patient may not need fluids when asleep, one cannot make this assumption unless the patient has been assessed. The patient is known to have poor fluid intake and may be dehydrated, therefore there is a chance that the patient will need the fluids. However, all of this cannot be assumed, and a clinical assessment needs to be done.

C - Give a verbal order to prescribe 0.9% Normal Saline 1L over 12 hours

It is dangerous to give a verbal order for any medication including IV fluids without first making an assessment of the patient. For example, this patient may be volume overloaded, hypernatraemic or not in need of IV fluids.

This is summarised in the following guidance:

'Prescribe drugs or treatment, including repeat prescriptions, only when you have adequate knowledge of the patient's health and are satisfied that the drugs or treatment serve the patient's needs.' (Good Medical Practice, paragraph 16a).

Question 17: Unwritten drug chart

In a busy Admissions Unit, patients are often moved before all documentation is complete making this scenario a common occurrence. A balance must be struck between fulfilling feelings of responsibility and respecting the handover system that is in place to ensure effective continuity of care. This scenario tests commitment to professionalism, coping with pressure, effective communication, patient focus, and working effectively within a team.

The correct order for this question is:

A.B.E.C.D.

A - Hand the task over to the night team

This is the most appropriate response as a good drug history is extremely important for patient safety and should not be rushed. It is also important not to delay such a task as the patient may be in need of his medication. As the patient is not acutely unwell, and you are at the end of your shift, a good drug history should be left for the night team to pursue. The following GMC guideline reflects the need for effective handover in modern shift based hospital work:

'You must contribute to the safe transfer of patients between healthcare providers...This means you must:

***a** share all relevant information with colleagues involved in your patients' care within and outside the team, including when you hand over care as you go off duty...'*

(Good Medical Practice, paragraph 44a).

B - Phone his next of kin to ask about his regular medication

Although one may be reluctant to make a call to the next of kin at midnight, patient safety should be the first priority. This option comes second as you are at the end of your shift and therefore shouldn't need to rush in gathering a good drug history.

E - Leave an entry in the notes for the day team/pharmacist to check with the GP the next morning

If neither the night team nor you are able to gather an adequate history, then it is important to effectively communicate the task over to the day team as emphasised by the above guidance. Leaving an entry in the notes can be an effective way of communicating this across, and for this reason option E is deemed more appropriate than C, where no measures have been taken to inform the day team of the patient's needs.

C - Write up some PRN (as needed) basic analgesia and leave it for the day team to find out the regular medications

This is a poor option as there is no indication for the patient to be placed on PRN analgesia, and this option also makes no attempt to hand the information over. However, it is more appropriate than option D where patient safety could potentially be placed at risk.

D - Look on the computer system for previous admissions and medications

This is potentially a dangerous approach to take, as there is a possibility that the patient's medications have changed since his last admission. For this reason, the medication list from a previous entry is not a suitable source of information to base a drug history for a patient.

Question 18: Self-discharge

This question is about assessing a precarious situation and acting decisively to prioritise your actions in order to minimise potential harm to the patient. The least desirable outcome is clearly for the patient to walk out of hospital with no further medical input whatsoever.

The correct order for this scenario is:

C.B.D.E.A.

C - Explain to the patient that a high potassium can cause dangerously abnormal heart rhythms

Hyperkalaemia is a medical emergency and can cause fatal arrythmias, in particular ventricular fibrillation. For this reason, the most important first step would be to explain this to the patient, which in turn may help solve his demands to self-discharge. Listening to the patient's concerns (B) is reasonable, however, one should not delay intervention when faced with such an emergency. He may be unaware that his potassium is raised and may even know about the potential complications of hyperkalaemia. His immediate co-operation is required to try and reduce the potassium levels. Medical knowledge of hyperkalaemia is required to answer this question, however, it is essential information to know and a common presentation to junior doctors.

B - Listen to the patient's concerns

Listening to the patient's concerns would be an appropriate next step in order to understand why he wants to leave, and in turn engaging in a discussion with him as to the necessity of his staying. This would be more appropriate than immediately seeking senior help, as a junior would not have reached the limitations of their capabilities by listening to a patient's concerns.

D - Call your senior colleague for advice

Having chosen options C and B one must reassess the scenario and consider the remaining options based on their own merit while ignoring the two options already chosen. For this reason, it would be most appropriate to seek senior advice when faced with such a situation before attempting to obtain a blood sample. A senior may be able to help you in advising the patient to remain in hospital, or if the patient still wishes to self-discharge then a senior colleague may be able to suggest options for making the discharge as safe as possible. If the patient no longer wishes to self-discharge then it would still be reasonable to seek advice from a senior colleague who may suggest initiating the appropriate management for hyperkalaemia.

E - Obtain a repeat blood sample

It is important to recheck the potassium, but the above options are more immediately important. If the patient self-discharges, then you will not be in a position to offer him any further assistance. Without communicating with the patient initially, a blood sample would be very difficult to obtain.

A - Offer him a 'discharge against medical advice' form and stress to him the importance of visiting his GP

Hyperkalaemia is an emergency and all appropriate measures should be taken to explain the importance of this to a patient. If however the patient is still adamant on leaving, then that is his choice (granted he has capacity) and must be respected. However, this is only after the risks and dangers have been thoroughly explained.

Question 19: Sick leave

Doctors can often be given new jobs while in the middle of many others and dealing with this appropriately and efficiently is essential. Signing sick leave forms is a common request and doctors must complete such requests or at least make the necessary arrangements to do so. This is clearly outlined in the New Doctor 2009 guidance:

'F1 doctors must:

be able to complete or arrange for the completion of legal documents correctly such as those certifying sickness and death (or arranging for these documents to be filled in) and liaise with the coroner or procurator fiscal where appropriate.'
(New Doctor 2009, paragraph 11b).

The correct order for this question is therefore:

C.A.D.B.E.

C - Tell the nurse you are still on the ward round and you will call the patient at home once discharged and post the sick leave form once the appropriate time has been decided by the team

On a busy firm with potentially many jobs to do, it is not appropriate to leave the ward round for a while and is also unfair on your colleagues, especially if it is only to fill in a sick leave form. However, sick leave forms must be completed and a clear plan to arrange the completion while you have other priorities is perfectly justifiable. This option ensures your decision is an informed one and you could explore issues that the patient may be worried about and their occupational status.

A - Tell the nurse that you have no time to explore further than what you already know about the patient and if the sick leave needs to be extended the patient can attend the GP surgery

If you are unable to arrange the sick leave form then you can ask the GP to review and make an informed decision. This is clearly a difficult decision to make and requires thought; as a laparoscopic procedure rarely requires 4 weeks for recovery, and therefore completion of the form should not be rushed.

D - Attend to the patient and complete the sick form accurately and return to the ward round as soon as possible, apologising to your team for your absence

This is a poorer option to take due to your current circumstances on the busy ward round. Only delay your urgent work if there is no other way to complete of the sick leave form. In this case, complete the form rapidly and apologise to your team to maintain professional integrity. It would be less detrimental to leave the ward round as there is another FY1 there, however, it is poor practice to leave ward rounds for non-urgent tasks as it disrupts the efficiency of your work.

B - Let the nurse know that sick leave authorisation is a doctor's decision

This option has a number of unfavourable outcomes. It firstly does not arrange any further exploration into the nurse's concerns and dismisses her suggestion unfairly. Furthermore, the tone of such a reply is not a good form of communication and can create problems within teams. Clearly the nurse is considering the best interests of the patient, therefore reasoning with the patient or arranging a plan of action for the nurse is a better option.

E - Sign the form for four weeks as the nurse seems confident in her decision and return to ward round

Although in many instances the decision made by nurses will be correct, doctors remain responsible for the duration of sick leave. Therefore, changing your clinical decision purely based on the nurse's suggestion is inappropriate, unless the reasoning is clearly communicated to you. You should be satisfied that what you are signing for is appropriate, and if not should take the relevant steps to ensuring it is.

Question 20: An angry pharmacist

The correct answers to this question are:

C.D.E.A.B.

C - Ask the daughter to return to the patient's bedside and you will come and speak with her shortly after reviewing the notes

This response shows the daughter of the patient that you are taking her concerns seriously, and also has the added effect of allowing her to calm down. This will give you time to compose yourself and approach the daughter with all the relevant information necessary to ascertain the source of her complaint. This is all the more important given that you have only taken over this patient's care a short while ago, so any conversation should be made with all the facts available. For these reasons, option C is preferred to option D, as it gives you time to review the patient's case and allows the relative time to calm down.

Additionally, the daughter's open hostility towards you in front of other staff members must not be a barrier to continuing to provide high quality care and treating the patient and her relative in a professional manner.

D - Review the drug chart and patient's notes to check whether or not any mention was made of an adverse reaction to Tramadol

This is to clarify whether there is any documented intolerance and whether Tramadol has been expressly mentioned previously. It is good practice to review the history of a new patient before speaking to their relative, even more so in the case of an angry relative. If it is apparent that there has been an oversight and the patient has been given Tramadol despite a clear warning in the notes or elsewhere, then an apology should be offered and steps taken to amend the mistake and prevent it from happening in the future.

'You must be open and honest with patients if things go wrong. If a patient under your care has suffered harm or distress, you should:

a put matters right (if that is possible)

b offer an apology

c explain fully and promptly what has happened and the likely short-term and long-term effects.'

(Good Medical Practice, paragraph 55).

E - Speak to your SHO about the situation

Advice from a senior can be very helpful in this situation. It may also help alleviate some of the anger of the patient's daughter as she can appreciate steps are being made to resolve the issue with the inclusion of senior clinicians. Your senior would also help guide and support you in this dialogue. However, the options above are preferable as they include taking initiative to deal with the situation yourself, before escalating to a senior.

A - Document the encounter in the patient's notes

It is important to document communication made with patients' relatives. This is especially the case when a patient threatens legal action. Every entry should be correctly dated and signed. It is also helpful to inform another colleague of the encounter and include their name in the entry as a witness to the discussions.

This option does not directly deal with the angry relative or the patient in the immediate time and therefore is not as appropriate as the answers above.

B - Tell the patient's daughter that you will not speak to her unless she calms down

This is likely to aggravate the daughter and exacerbate the situation. Angry relatives and patients should be listened to and respected in order to help rectify the problem. This, of course, does not mean they can be abusive or aggressive towards health professionals. However, allowing relatives to air their grievances often helps them calm down and helps towards resolving a tense situation.

'You must be considerate to those close to the patient, and be sensitive and responsive in giving them information and support.' (Good Medical Practice, paragraph 33).

Question 21: You want my honest opinion?

It is always important to give honest and constructive feedback to students following a task. This is important in improving their skills and therefore benefitting patients in the long term. It is vital to let a student know where they went wrong if you believe they have. At the same time it is also important not to be so antagonising with your feedback that the student loses confidence and feels belittled. This is summarised within the following GMC guidance:

'You must be honest and objective when writing references, and when appraising or assessing the performance of colleagues, including locums and students.' (Good Medical Practice, paragraph 41).

This would make the following options most appropriate:

D.E.H.

D - Ask him to come back later this week and perform the examination again for the signature

E - Encourage him to reflect on his examination and refuse to sign

H - Offer him material to read up on but don't sign

In this scenario, it is important that you do not sign the logbook based on the reasons and guidelines above. Therefore, as well as these answers, option B is also in keeping with the rationale of refusing to sign. However, option B is the harsher of the options and while it may serve as a wake up call to some students, it may also diminish confidence in others and be upsetting. Option D is a fair approach to take and is realistic, giving the student time to read up on the technique and try again. Option E illustrates a vitally important tool for students and doctors of all stages to apply throughout their career; reflection. After performing a task, a period of time spent in reflection enables one to think about how one might approach the situation differently in the future and what one might change. Reflection can also occur via discussion with other colleagues, and this technique in general helps a person improve on performances and helps close the gap of 'unknown unknowns', as explained within the Johari window concept. Option H is, practically speaking, a very useful option for the student and is definitely a reasonable approach to take.

While option A is somewhat honest, it still conflicts with the GMC guidance and is unhelpful to the student who will feel his examination was good enough. Likewise, option C is unhelpful towards the student and can provide false hope for him come exam time! Option F is inappropriate and should not be used as a means of signing logbooks. Although option G is reasonable, it does, however, involve speaking through the examination as opposed to performing it as was required for the signature. Furthermore, there is a big difference between clinically performing an examination and talking through it, with the former being more relevant to medical practice.

Question 22: Capacity versus confidentiality?

Mental capacity is assessed by a patient being able to understand, retain, weigh up and communicate information related to making a decision. A note to make is that mental capacity is relative to the decision being made, for example a person deemed not to have mental capacity for making medical decisions may still be able to choose their lunch. It is important to understand how to deal with situations when a patient without mental capacity insists on making autonomous decisions on matters related to their health. The principle of beneficence must be maintained, as recognised by the maxim *'Salus aegroti suprema lex'* - The well-being of the patient is the most important law. In this scenario, it would be appropriate to discuss the patient's condition with the daughter as it would be in her best interest, as outlined by the following GMC guideline:

'If a patient who lacks capacity asks you not to disclose personal information about their condition or treatment, you should try to persuade them to allow an appropriate person to be involved in the consultation. If they refuse, and you are convinced that it is essential in their best interests, you may disclose relevant information to an appropriate person or authority...' *(Confidentiality, paragraph 61).*

The most suitable options to take in this scenario would be:

A.F.H.

A - Arrange a convenient time to discuss the patient's condition with her daughter

F - Apologetically reject the patient's wishes

H - Explain to the patient that you will need to disclose information and write your reasons for doing so in the notes

The scenario clearly communicates that the patient has 'advanced Alzheimer's Disease' and is 'deemed not to have mental capacity to make decisions on her health'. It also states that the patient is being treated for an 'acute severe asthma attack'. Thus, not involving next of kin in such circumstances would pose significant challenges in effectively managing the patient's condition. Input from family members would be vital to record a good medical history, understand the patient's social circumstances and plan safe discharge. These reasons make options A and F favourable and correct. Furthermore, the scenario does not suggest that there are problems in the daughter–mother relationship, in which case, further evaluation of whether a disclosure of the patient's clinical information may have been warranted.

Option H is also very important. For effective communication with other members of staff as well as for medico-legal reasons, it is always important to document verbal agreements made with patients to avoid any confusion and misunderstanding in the future.

Option B adopts a crude tone and is inconsiderate to the patient's feelings. It is also not true that a patient cannot make 'any decisions' as mental capacity is relative, as discussed above. Option C is not in the patient's best interests and it is important that her condition is discussed with the daughter, as has been justified above. Option D alludes to the fact that you also won't be disclosing information to the daughter, and is therefore an inappropriate approach to take. Option E, similarly to option B, demonstrates a lack of respect towards the patient, and this should always be avoided, especially in the care of vulnerable patients. Option G is an ineffective approach to take, as the patient has already been deemed not to have mental capacity, and thus, the option of disclosure does not rest on her decision, rather on the principle of beneficence being applied.

Question 23: A laxative mistake

Your GMC registration number is given to you shortly after qualifying and remains the same throughout your career. It is a GMC principle that when asked for your number, you should make it available:

'If someone you have contact with in your professional role asks for your registered name and/or GMC reference number, you must give this information to them.' (Good Medical Practice, paragraph 64).

Mistakes can occur in hospital and it is important to be sensitive to patient views even if you are not at fault. A patient deserves to be listened to and given an explanation when something goes wrong, as summarised below:

'You must respond promptly, fully and honestly to complaints and apologise when appropriate. You must not allow a patient's complaint to adversely affect the care or treatment you provide or arrange.' (Good Medical Practice, paragraph 61).

Combining both of these principles, the most appropriate options to take would be:

A.D.F.

A - Explain to the patient that you did not prescribe the laxatives but will help find out who it was

D - Reluctantly give the patient your name and number whilst informing him of your innocence

F - Take the patient into a quiet room to explore his concerns

Option A helps clarify to the patient that it was not you who prescribed the laxatives. This may or may not help in reducing his level of frustration, however, it does establish a level of mutual understanding from which you can build upon. In this option you go on to offer your assistance to address some of the patient's concerns, and this may help diffuse some of the patient's anger. Option D is in keeping with the guidance mentioned above, and while you may be reluctant to hand your number over after being wrongly accused, it is also important to inform the patient of the situation to the best of your knowledge as the option suggests. Option F is an essential technique in communicating with patients, and where possible should not be neglected. Pursuing this path will make the patient feel that his concerns are being taken seriously, increase his confidence in the doctor-patient relationship, and help resolve the situation.

While some of the actions taken in option B are correct, the approach adopted is incorrect. Making demands on the patient, especially as he has legitimate grievances, may anger the patient further and lead to an escalation of the situation. Option C is unnecessary in this scenario and could further frustrate the patient who has every right to be distressed at the team for the mistake. Option E does not deal with the situation, avoids the problem and is unprofessional. Option G may seem reasonable, however, this focuses on defending your innocence rather than dealing with the patient's current distress, and so relative to the answers selected, is not as appropriate. Option H is in contradiction with the GMC guidelines and is not an open and constructive response to take.

Question 24: Ditched by your SHO

The correct answers to this scenario are: **B.D.F.**

B - Speak to your registrar about the situation

D - Disagree with your SHO and insist he shares the workload

F - Speak to the SHO on the other team about the situation

Option B is a good approach, and is superior to option C as stepwise approach must be taken when escalating issues to senior colleagues. If your SHO is not willing to listen to your concerns, informing your registrar would be an appropriate step to take. From the scenario, it appears that you have already attempted to 'discuss the situation with your SHO' but he still doesn't seem willing to sympathise with your distress. While he may agree to help on this occasion, he appears to have the wrong attitude and therefore a discussion with the registrar on the team is appropriate and has the potential to yield good results.

You should nevertheless continue to make it clear that you need the SHO's help (D). Patient care must be your priority. It is also not fair on yourself that you are finding it difficult to stay on top of your work as you have to work alone. In this instance, where the conduct of a colleague is affecting the care you provide patients:

'You must take prompt action if you think that patient safety, dignity or comfort is or may be seriously compromised.' (Good Medical Practice paragraph 25).

Challenging a senior colleague can be very difficult and is something that must be approached with great care so as not to damage the working relationship.

'You should challenge colleagues if their behaviour does not comply with this guidance, and follow the guidance in paragraph 25c if the behaviour amounts to abuse of a patient's or colleague's rights.' (Good Medical Practice paragraph 59)

Seeking the advice of another SHO would be helpful, both in terms of helping you in your approach to the situation, and also because it is possible that another SHO could directly advise your SHO about the situation and he may be more receptive to the advice (F).

(A & E & H) These options are not acceptable as they have the potential to adversely affect good patient care. They also do not address the fundamental problem in this scenario, and result in the continuation of this ongoing problem. Option A will add to your levels of stress and work load, and thus negatively impact on how well you are able to deliver care to your patients. Besides not addressing the issue, option E can also have adverse affects on patient care if duties beyond the medical student's competencies are designated to her. Option H causes a new problem by inappropriately overburdening the on-call team with your routine ward jobs.

(C) This would not be appropriate as a first response to the problem because there are other avenues that have not yet been explored. A possible drawback from this approach would be the SHO feeling undermined and upset that you went directly to the consultant before discussing the matter further with him or the registrar. Furthermore, the word 'complain' is not ideal in this option and would not be the best approach to take to the consultant. One should escalate appropriately based on the circumstance. GMC guidelines state:

'If you have reason to believe that patients are, or may be, at risk of death of serious harm for any reason, you should report your concern to the appropriate person or organisation immediately...such as the consultant in charge of the team...'

The scenario would not warrant immediate escalation to the consultant, rather, it is an issue which juniors should be able to resolve amongst themselves.

Option G aims to direct the ward jobs towards the SHO. This does not affect the fundamental problem at hand. It is also likely that the SHO may redirect these jobs towards you, and thus you would be back at 'square one'.

Question 25: Challenging the SHO's decision?

Working effectively in a team and providing the best patient care can be difficult at times. This case illustrates this in a difficult scenario that focuses on areas of care of vulnerable patients, professionalism, medical acumen, communication and teamwork. With this in mind the correct answers are:

B.E.G.

B - Ask the SHO to examine the patient properly while still at the bed side

E - After the ward round, tell the SHO, clearly and assertively, that you refuse to document false information about patients

G - Apologise to the patient and explore her concerns

It is worthwhile noting that many answer options in this scenario are quite harsh, thus you are required to distinguish between these answers and select the most appropriate ones. The most effective way to resolve the problem is to ask your SHO to examine the patient, as is expected from a junior doctor. This is especially relevant as patients who have dementia do not always have the ability to voice their concerns. Furthermore, patients who are declared to be 'medically fit' may develop subsequent medical problems. Asking your SHO to examine the patient (B) will resolve the problem of inaccurate and false documentation. It is important to remember that the feedback should be verbalised in a non-confrontational manner using effective communication skills. Option G works in tandem, as you are seeking to find out if the patient has any problems. As there is a disagreement happening, this may become apparent to the patient, and putting the patient at ease by apologising is also commendable. Both these options serve the best interests of the patient. Option E does come across as harsh, and ideally, should be done politely; however, relative to the other remaining options; it is preferred. It is important that you openly and directly deal with this matter, and clarify your position. This will help prevent similar occurrences in the future, and it may also serve as useful feedback to the SHO.

Answer A is plausible as you should not write anything unless it is accurate and honest. Therefore, refusal to do so is understandable but does not resolve the primary problem of ensuring the proper care of a vulnerable patient and the potential of untruthful documentation. Intending to confront your SHO about the unprofessional and unsafe practice away from the patient is professional and considerate. The GMC advise:

'*19* Documents you make (including clinical records) to formally record your work must be clear, accurate and legible. You should make records at the same time as the events you are recording or as soon as possible afterwards.'

'*21* Clinical records should include:

a relevant clinical findings

b the decisions made and actions agreed, and who is making the decisions and agreeing the actions

c the information given to patients

d any drugs prescribed or other investigation or treatment work is making the record and when.'

(Good Medical Practice, paragraphs 19 and 21).

Option C is a poor option as it is very confrontational, lacks insight into effective teamwork, and is also inconsiderate of your own clinical limitations (the scenario mentions that this is your first week on the firm). This option is likely to result in an active conflict with your SHO, and make the problem greater than what it was.

Option H is inappropriate as incorrect documentation is being made and this contradicts probity and proper patient care.

Leaving the ward round is not a professional means to deal with this problem and you should make efforts to always resolve issues with effective communication skills. Furthermore, this will not ensure better patient safety for this patient and compromises patient care for the other patients who you will not attend to. The New Doctor 2009 document suggests an FY1 should strive to:

'Work effectively as a member of a team, including supporting others, handover and taking over the care of a patient safely and effectively from other health professionals.' (New doctors, paragraph 10a).

Answer F is not recommended at this stage as you should first discuss the situation with the SHO directly, and only if this does not lead to the resolution of the problem, you should consider escalating.

Question 26: Ward round prescribing

This answer highlights the importance of recognising potential emergencies and the importance of prompt apologies to patients when an error is made.

The three best options in this scenario are:

B.C.D.

B - Call microbiology for advice on alternative therapy

C - Attend to the patient and ensure she is clinically stable

D - Explain to the patient why this error has occurred

As this is a potentially hazardous scenario, the care of your patient must be your first concern and therefore option C is very important. This course of action allows the immediate assessment of the situation, especially in case your patient goes into an anaphylactic shock. This is clearly not an assessment that a nurse should be responsible for as option A proposes.

Of the options left, the next priority after the primary assessment remains to apologise to the patient promptly as per guidance (Good Medical Practice, paragraph 55).

Therefore, option D is clearly justifiable and the patient should be aware of the potential risk she faces. This may result in a negative reaction from the patient and a complaint but this is not a reason to avoid an apology and explanation. It has been reported repeatedly in the medico-legal literature that a prompt and sincere apology reduced the likelihood of complaints. The GMC encourages apologising to complaining patients where appropriate:

'You must respond promptly, fully and honestly to complaints and apologise when appropriate. You must not allow a patient's complaint to adversely affect the care or treatment you provide or arrange.' (Good Medical Practice, paragraph 61).

Option B works very well with options C and D, and helps optimise care by changing the antibiotics to an appropriate alternative. This will also make the discussion with the patient easier, as you have an alternative management plan ready to address her clinical issues.

Option E, to call the registrar, is incorrect relative to the other options, as the initial assessment has to be made first and you should try and address any immediate needs before calling your seniors.

Option F is a poor option, as there is a clear cause of the rash. It would be premature to ask for a dermatology review at this stage.

Option G and H are both good courses of action to adopt, however, are not the most appropriate actions in this scenario. Once the needs of the patient are resolved, an incident form should be completed, and an audit may be performed. It would be premature to prioritise these actions above those that are aimed at redressing the mistake and optimising the care of the patient in question. A small delay in submitting the incident form or the audit proposal will not make much of a difference; in contrast, delaying options B/C/D can have significant negative consequences.

Question 27: On call and unresponsive!

Similar scenarios commonly present in practice and the time available to prioritise your thoughts can be minimal, therefore having a good idea of what is important is essential. In all cases, it is crucial to '*make the care of your patient your first concern*'. Therefore, in a scenario like this, one must take into account the guidance below:

'You must offer help if emergencies arise in clinical settings or in the community, taking account of your own safety, your competence and the availability of other options for care.' (Good Medical Practice, paragraph 26).

C.D.F.

C - Ask the nurse to use the SBAR* tool for the handover of information

D - Leave the patient you are reviewing and attend to the new patient

F - Tell the nurse that her request is very poorly communicated

The first priority is patient safety and therefore, establishing a clear understanding of what is going on is vital. By doing this, you are able to not only risk stratify the patient, but also offer advice over the phone that may be necessary and urgent. The best way to do this as established in UK practice is through a systematic method such as the SBAR tool described in option C, or a similar effective communication tool. It also makes it clear to the nurse that you are not asking for unnecessary details. In balancing the needs of the two patients within the scenario, your current patient is said to be 'stable' while the nurse's patient seems to be 'unresponsive'. For this reason, it would be appropriate to attend to the nurse's patient despite the little information provided by her due to the clinical need (D), as opposed to continuing your review of the stable patient (A). Option F is a justifiable response to her abrupt enquiry, and has potential to facilitate the acquisition of further information. Basic information will help you in formulating possible diagnoses/investigation and management plans as you rush off to review the patient, and also gives you the opportunity to offer the nurse advice in the meantime until you arrive. It is true that the nurse may respond negatively to such a statement, however, when weighing up the potential benefits of highlighting her error and re-enforcing the need for more information (C), this option is relatively superior to all the other remaining options.

If, as may be likely in this scenario, the nurse does not offer you any further details, then a threat of unwillingness to see the patient is inappropriate, due to the potential harm that could result to the nurse's patient (B). Inviting the nurse to make a medical emergency team call or start resuscitation based on the patient 'seeming' to be unresponsive, as in option E, is not appropriate with the little information you have. There can be many causes to a patient 'seeming unresponsive' and importantly you are not even aware of the patient's DNAR (Do Not Attempt Resuscitation) status. Nurses are fully aware of how to make a 'crash call' and when it should be made. Bleeping the registrar (G) in such a situation is inappropriate and does not use initiative, as this is a situation where a junior doctor should be able to make an assessment of the situation and instigate management before escalation to seniors. As always, filing an incident form (H) is a plausible response, but should be done at a later time when the problem is resolved. It improves care for future patients but does not help care for the current patient who may be in urgent need of help.

Question 28: The 'crash-call' relative

This is a difficult scenario for a number of reasons. Firstly this is a true life and death scenario that requires the utmost focus and attention of all members of the arrest team. It is also a highly emotive situation, with a patient dying and a relative outside feeling helpless.

The correct answers are:

A.E.G.

A - Politely refuse the husband's request to observe the unfolding events

E - Ask the sister in charge to explain to the husband that his wife is critical and that every attempt to resuscitate her is being made

G - Inform the sister in charge that you'd like to have a thorough discussion with the husband later

(A) Having the husband in the background may act as a distraction to some of the team members, thus preventing them from directing their full attention to the patient. The patient's husband has most likely never seen his wife attached to multiple drips and monitors, while someone is performing chest compressions. This is a very distressing sight, and is likely to evoke a very strong emotional response. The scenario mentions that you have reached the fourth cycle of CPR and that the prognosis is poor, thus it is likely that a team discussion regarding stopping the resuscitation efforts will be required soon. Such a discussion will be made even more difficult if the husband was to be present. It would therefore be better for the husband not to observe the arrest in this scenario.

Option E is very important, as a senior member of staff is explaining the situation to the husband, and reassuring him that every effort is being made to resuscitate his wife. This will increase his faith in the team carrying out the resuscitation effort, and also enable him to understand why he is being prevented from attending to his wife at this very point in time.

Option G is an appropriate course of action to take as it seeks to reassure the husband that the doctor will sit down with him and provide him with all the relevant information. It also reinforces to him that the primary focus remains on the resuscitation effort, which is the reason why the doctor cannot update him now.

As the team leader of a resuscitation attempt into its fourth cycle, you should remain on the scene in order to ensure everything is well coordinated, as opposed to leaving the arrest to update the husband yourself (F).

(C) It is important to involve members of the team in decisions, especially when it may potentially affect their own performance. However, in such an emergency it would act as an obvious distraction to 'discuss' such a request with the other members, and one's full focus should be on resuscitating the patient at this time. A resuscitation attempt requires a synchronised effort from all team members which can only come about with undivided attention at all times.

While it may not necessarily be wrong to opt for option D, the explanation for option A has explained why it is highly unfavourable, and this option has not been selected.

(H) The husband deserves a thorough explanation of the circumstance, and a discussion 'through the curtain' will not provide the husband the information he is seeking. This approach also diverts one's attention from the arrest and is therefore not a good step to take.

'You must be considerate to those close to the patient, and be sensitive and responsive in giving them information and support.' (Good Medical Practice, paragraph 33).

(B) There are no definitive formal guidelines provided by the resuscitation council about family members attending a resuscitation attempt. The guidelines mention the different advantages and disadvantages of having family members present at an arrest call, however, no absolute action is advised in this regard. Each situation is unique, and requires the doctor to use his/her clinical experience, communication skills and empathy to make a judgement that is appropriate to the scenario. While this option is reasonable, in the acute setting described in the scenario, it does not address the husband's needs as directly as the other options. He will understandably be distressed and not in a suitable state to wait for the sister to 'try and find any local guidelines'.

Question 29: Prioritising your workload

An all too familiar situation: juggling an already busy workload when an extra demand is placed on you. This scenario, as well as being about prioritising, is also about not forgetting your duty of care to your patients.

B.E.F.

B - Inform your team that you are needed in theatre

E - Consult your jobs list and delegate any jobs that are urgent

F - Tell your on-call FY1 colleague that he's needed in theatre and to take over from you once he has finished lunch

(B & E) The first step should be to see what jobs you have to do for the patients who are under your care. You must ensure that there are no urgent tasks that are required for any of these patients. You must inform your team that you will be in theatre and ask for their permission. There is nothing mentioned in the scenario to indicate that you are very busy, and you have already offered to assist your colleague, thus you should make a reasonable effort to assist your colleague in this circumstance.

(F)You should inform your on-call FY1 colleague that he is needed in theatre, and make sure that he knows he needs to relieve you as you must return to the ward. However, in this instance, providing your team are happy with you going to theatre, you are assisting your colleague as well as ensuring that none of your own clinical duties are being neglected. This is a wise approach as you are planning ahead.

(C) It may be possible to find another FY1 to cover you, but only after you have given them a thorough handover of all your jobs and patients. The tendency in this situation would be to perhaps rush a handover to make it to theatre. It is preferred to keep the jobs for your ward within the team who already know the patients and therefore, will require little handover information, as outlined in options B and E.

Options A and G are on either end of the spectrum, with option A being neglectful to the registrar's needs in theatre, and option G being neglectful to your own ward duties. Seeing as the bleep has just gone off within a couple of minutes, it would not be appropriate to call your colleague back and ask him to go to theatre (D), having just agreed to hold his bleep for 30 minutes. You understand that he is tired as outlined in the scenario and so it would be best to find alternative avenues to deal with the situation before pressuring him to go to theatre. While option H makes sense in theory, practically it should not matter how long the surgery is as you can swap with a colleague at any time during the procedure. What dictates your decision should be your current workload (B, E) as well as the availability of your colleague once back from his lunch break (F).

Question 30: The battle for annual leave

To ensure adequate hospital staffing levels, all annual leave requests has to be approved by the rota co-ordinator. Furthermore, if there are any on-call commitments that have been swapped, the rota coordinator must be fully informed. If the rota coordinator does not know of the swap, then the responsibility of the on-call duty remains with the doctor originally allocated to work the shift.

The most appropriate responses are:

A.D.G.

A - Ask the rota coordinator whether she can arrange a locum doctor to work the weekend in question

D - Try and find a FY1 from another specialty to work your weekend and work a weekend of his/her choice in return

G - Arrange a meeting with the leave coordinator and the FY1 with whom you had swapped the shift

(D) The ideal action would be to find another doctor who is able to work the medical shift providing they have the right skills to do this. This would ensure that your holiday plans are not affected, and would also satisfy the staffing needs.

(G) A compromise may be reached if the leave coordinator, who is used to dealing with these situations regularly, and the FY1 doctor in question, arrange to meet to discuss the issue and explore available options.

(A) This is not ideal, but is relatively more superior to all the remaining options. Here, you are suggesting a viable (yet expensive) alternative, for the rota coordinator to consider. Whether the coordinator decides to accept or refuse your request is up to him/her, however, your request is not unreasonable in light of your particular circumstances.

(E) If no one can be found, you may have to curtail your holiday to fulfil your on-call commitments. Occasionally medical staffing will provide locum cover, but in return you may be expected to work another weekend of their choosing. This option has not been selected here, as it is important that you explore all possible avenues before you change your holiday plans (which will incur extra expenses upon you, and will leave you disgruntled).

'Check, where practical, that a named clinician or team has taken over responsibility when your role in providing a patient's care has ended.' (Good Medical Practice, paragraph 44b).

(C) One must never claim to be sick so he/she can take leave. This action would seriously call into question the individual's probity.

'You must make sure that your conduct justifies your patients' trust in you and the public's trust in the profession.' (Good Medical Practice, paragraph 65).

(H) You have a duty of care to your patients and cannot leave an unfilled gap in the rota. In this option, you are neglecting the issue at hand, which could lead to a gap in the rota, and adversely affect patient care. Furthermore, the swap was 'informal' and therefore you are responsible for finding suitable cover.

(F) It is not possible for a replacement FY1 from another trust to work your on-call. This doctor is not known to your trust, and needs to be first approved by the human recourses department. Only an approved locum may work the weekend shift. You should not seek to cover your shifts externally, bypassing the proper channels, however well intentioned the offer may be.

Practice Paper

2

Questions

Question 1: Just hours before the operation begins

You are on a busy medical ward and are looking after a patient who has been admitted for an elective ERCP scheduled for the following day. The patient is due to have platelets administered one hour prior to the procedure tomorrow. However, you incorrectly prescribe fresh frozen plasma. On the day of the procedure, you realise your mistake and contact the laboratory who inform you that the platelets need to be obtained from another hospital and will not be available until the next day. The patient is due to have his ERCP in a few hours time.

Rank in order the following actions in response to this situation (1= Most appropriate; 5= Least appropriate)

a) Explain to the patient that due to technical difficulties in the lab, his ERCP has been delayed

b) Apologise to the patient for your mistake and explain that the ERCP will be delayed

c) Ask the nursing staff to go and speak to the patient regarding the mistake

d) Bleep your registrar and inform him of the situation

e) Inform the laboratory of the situation and ask them to consider ordering urgent platelets before the planned ERCP on the day

Question 2: Nutritional treatment over medications

A 66 year old vegan patient is admitted with acute asthma. She has clinically improved and is now ready for discharge. When writing her discharge letter, you notice that her capillary blood glucose samples were persistently very high (15-20mmol) and that a number of blood tests done over admission suggest diabetes. The patient believes this is due to her diet of sugary fruits and pulses and doesn't want to have any medical investigations or treatment for diabetes whatsoever. She is keen to be discharged today as she has 'had it up to here' with being in hospital.

Rank in order the following actions in response to this situation (1= Most appropriate; 5= Least appropriate)

a) Respect her wishes and complete her discharge summary

b) Discuss the complications of diabetes with her

c) Inform the patient of the importance of eating a healthy balanced diet, including meat, to ward off other diet-related conditions

d) Offer her a review by the diabetic team as an outpatient

e) Inform the patient that you think she should remain in hospital for routine monitoring as that would be in her best interests

Question 3: Nobody likes a bully

You see your fellow renal FY1 in tears on a Monday morning. Speaking to her, it becomes clear that she is finding it very difficult to work with her SpR (Specialist Registrar), who she says is extremely demanding and likes picking up on every possible error. She tells you that despite her best efforts and even after repeatedly staying beyond her shift to ensure completion of all tasks, she still finds him unreasonably demanding. She says that she now hates coming into work, however, is worried that if she raises this issue she'll have an even more difficult time with him. You are also aware of other members of staff who have had problems working with this particular registrar.

Rank in order *the following actions in response to this situation (1= Most appropriate; 5= Least appropriate)*

a) Advise your colleague to talk to the registrar and explain how she feels

b) Suggest to your colleague that she takes some annual leave as it will help refresh her

c) Tell your colleague to raise this issue with the consultant

d) Ask her to email the foundation programme director

e) Tell her to persevere with him as it is not just her who finds him difficult, and she is only there for three more months

Question 4: Anxious relatives

During the morning ward round, the consultant asks you to discharge a patient with ulcerative colitis after he claims that he is feeling well. In the afternoon, the nurses inform you that the family are unhappy upon hearing of the decision to discharge and claim the patient is not being honest about his symptoms. They wish to speak to the consultant.

Rank in order *the following actions in response to this situation (1= Most appropriate; 5= Least appropriate)*

a) Ask the nurses to reassure the family that the consultant has reviewed the patient and he is fit for discharge

b) Contact the consultant

c) Discharge the patient as per the consultant's plan and ask him to re-attend if there are any concerns

d) Speak to the family about their concerns

e) Return to the patient in order to reassess his symptoms

Question 5: The referral bleep

You are working as an FY1 on the surgical assessment unit. The surgical registrar that takes the surgical referrals on the unit asks you to hold the referral bleep 'just for 30 minutes' while he takes a quick break. The referral bleep is how A&E doctors and GPs refer to the surgical team at your hospital. It is 4.30pm and the registrar has not had a break since he started at 9am. You know it is hospital policy that only the surgical registrar takes referrals.

Rank in order the following actions in response to this situation *(1= Most appropriate; 5= Least appropriate)*

a) Agree and tell the registrar not to rush, you feel capable and want to help your colleague

b) Reluctantly agree and inform your consultant of the registrar's irresponsible actions once the registrar returns

c) Decline to hold the bleep as you are not authorised, and help him contact someone suitable (another surgical registrar)

d) Decline to hold the bleep saying it's against the rules and you never get breaks

e) Accept the bleep and inform everyone who bleeps that you cannot accept or decline referrals but will take the details

Question 6: Second Opinion

A family member of a patient who is being managed by another team approaches you regarding the DNAR (Do Not Attempt Resuscitation) status of her relative. She feels that the other team has given up hope on the patient and have inappropriately given the patient the DNAR status without proper consultation. She asks you to review the patient and asks your advice about the suitability of the decision.

Rank in order *the following actions in response to this situation (1= Most appropriate; 5= Least appropriate)*

a) Review the patient and discuss the suitability of the DNAR status

b) Contact the relevant team and inform them of the family's concerns

c) Inform the patient's family that you are not the patient's doctor and cannot alter the decision

d) Explore the family's concerns with them

e) Put a temporary hold on the DNAR status until you have had a discussion with the other team

Question 7: Off home at five on the dot

You are finishing up for the day when your registrar calls you aside. She informs you in an aggressive tone that it is not fair for the FY1 to leave at 5pm when the rest of the team, who are your seniors, are staying to complete the remaining jobs for the day. She informs you that repeatedly leaving at 5pm has upset other members of the team as well.

Rank in order the following actions in response to this situation *(1= Most appropriate; 5= Least appropriate)*

a) Inform the registrar that you were unaware that there were jobs left and offer to stay behind and help to complete those jobs

b) Explain that you are not obliged to stay beyond 5pm as those are your contracted hours

c) Explain that you have completed the jobs assigned to you for the day and it is not your responsibility to do other people's jobs for them

d) Apologise and speak to your clinical supervisor about this incident

e) Apologise and speak to your SHOs about this issue and clarify the expectations the team has of one another

Question 8: Third year wrestles with a cannula

While on your ward, you are called over by a nurse regarding a patient of yours, Mr. Smith. The nurse asks that you help the 'student doctor' who is trying to cannulate the patient. You go to the patient and find a third year medical student attempting to cannulate the patient for the third time. The patient and her relative are distressed. The student informs you that he overheard a nurse saying the patient needed a new cannula and thought he would try and insert one. He states that the nurse helped him find the equipment.

Rank in order *the following actions in response to this situation (1= Most appropriate; 5= Least appropriate)*

a) Inform the nurse in charge of the patient that students are not allowed to cannulate without permission and that in future the doctor should be told in the first instance if it appears that a student is preparing to perform one

b) Apologise to the patient for the failed attempts and insert the cannula yourself

c) Take the student aside and explain that he is not to attempt medical procedures without permission

d) Commend the student for his initiative and supervise him in attempting the cannula again

e) Inform the matron of this incident so that all staff members are made aware in order to prevent this happening in the future

Question 9: ABG from the wrong patient!

You arrive 10 minutes late for a post-take ward round. The first patient has already been seen. Your SHO informs you that the patient needs an ABG and asks you to perform it now. In your haste to catch up with the ward round, you inadvertently take an ABG from the patient in the bed next to the intended patient. You only realise this error when you return to the ward, after analysing the ABG sample, and a nurse asks about the results. In the meantime, the patient from whom you took the ABG is also keen to know the results.

Rank in order *the following actions in response to this situation (1= Most appropriate; 5= Least appropriate)*

a) Apologise to the patient you have taken the ABG from and explain that it was an unnecessary procedure

b) Take the ABG from the correct patient

c) Fill out a clinical incident form and inform your senior team member of what has happened

d) Keep the incident to yourself, as it has not caused any real harm to anyone

e) Discuss the incident with your clinical supervisor

Question 10: A Stressed SHO

It is your first week as an FY1. During a busy on-call, you receive a call from your SHO. She informs you that she is inundated with acutely unwell patients and has been asked to review two more. She asks that you review the first one. She provides you with a brief history and basic observations. You immediately feel that this patient sounds too complex for you to assess. The SHO sounds very stressed on the phone and asks you to bleep her once you have reviewed the patient, but warns it may be a while until she can come and see the patient, and that she trusts you to be able to perform a basic initial assessment.

Rank in order *the following actions in response to this situation (1= Most appropriate; 5= Least appropriate)*

a) Tell your SHO you do not feel comfortable seeing this patient alone

b) Review the patient and then call the registrar and inform him of the situation, and ask for advice

c) Review the patient and ensure that he/she is stable, then bleep the SHO to confirm your plan

d) Ask the nurses looking after the patient for advice

e) Offer to help the SHO with her current patients so that she can go and review this new patient

Question 11: Doctor in the family

When walking through the ward one afternoon, you notice the relative of one of your patients standing by the patient notes trolley. He is reading through the notes of his father who is a patient under your care. When confronted, he states that he is a qualified doctor from another hospital and can look at patient notes. He then proceeds to ask questions regarding the team's current management plan and insists on certain investigations being performed.

Rank in order the following actions in response to this situation *(1= Most appropriate; 5= Least appropriate)*

a) Inform the nurse in charge of the incident

b) Ask your registrar to come down to the ward and speak to the relative

c) Inform the relative that despite being a qualified doctor, he has no right to look through patient notes in this hospital

d) Explain to the relative that it is the responsibility of the team in charge of the patient to decide what investigations are needed

e) Document the encounter in the patient's notes

Question 12: The cannula in a cardiac arrest

You are the medical foundation year doctor on-call and are part of the resuscitation team. Your bleep alerts you to a cardiac arrest in one of the renal wards. When you arrive, the registrar (team leader) is reading through the notes, the anaesthetist is trying to secure the airway and the senior house officer is doing the chest compressions. The team leader asks you to gain intravenous access by inserting a large bore cannula, as the patient currently does not have access. You do not feel confident in inserting a large bore cannula as you have not done it before.

Rank in order the following actions in response to this situation (1= Most appropriate; 5= Least appropriate)

a) Offer to take an arterial blood gas sample instead

b) Insert a smaller sized cannula instead – after all access is access

c) Voice your concerns to the team leader

d) Attempt to insert a large bore cannula

e) Wait for the anaesthetist to insert a cannula after securing the airway

Question 13: The difficult arterial blood gas

You are in A&E clerking a patient who is known to have chronic obstructive pulmonary disease (COPD) and is on home oxygen and nebulisers.

Your history and examination conclude a differential diagnosis of infective exacerbation of COPD. Bloods have been taken, an intravenous cannula inserted, and treatment prescribed.

You are required to take an arterial blood gas, the patient states that this is his least favourite blood test but luckily he has been told that he is 'easy to get' and hence consents. You attempt twice and unfortunately fail. You attempt a third time, however, the analysis of the sample shows that it is a venous sample.

Rank in order *the following actions in response to this situation (1= Most appropriate; 5= Least appropriate)*

a) Apologise to the patient and ask if he would prefer for someone else to try

b) Call your senior house officer and ask her to try

c) Leave it and await registrar review as the pH is stable

d) Ask the surgical house officer on-call to attempt an ABG for you

e) Ask the on-call registrar for further advice

Question 14: Coping with a heavy workload

You are the house officer on a very busy medical firm. Currently, the senior house officer is on nights; but even when the full team is present, you have noted that you are always working through lunch, arriving late to the weekly compulsory foundation year teaching and leaving work late. You feel that you prioritise well and work hard, but you cannot see the situation changing in the near future.

Rank in order *the following actions in response to this situation (1= Most appropriate; 5= Least appropriate)*

a) Discuss the situation with your consultant

b) Reflect upon why you are taking too long to complete your tasks

c) Discuss the situation with medical staffing and demand that a locum senior house officer is brought in

d) Ask your registrar if you can leave at least fifteen minutes earlier on your teaching days

e) Discuss the situation with your educational supervisor, as you cannot see the situation changing

Question 15: Fatal potassium levels

You are the surgical house officer looking after an elderly gentleman with a history of mild cognitive impairment and metastatic colon cancer. He has developed bilateral hydronephrosis and renal failure due to obstruction of his ureters and has been admitted to the urology ward for placement of ureteric stents. The nurse has called you to see him as he is refusing to have the procedure; she also informs you that his most recent potassium result was 7.8 mmol/L. His ECG now shows changes consistent with hyperkalaemia.

Rank in order the following actions in response to this situation (1= Most appropriate; 5= Least appropriate)

a) Explain to the patient that he cannot refuse treatment that is in his best interests

b) Assess the patient's capacity to understand the advantages and disadvantages of the procedure

c) Listen to the patient's concerns about the procedure

d) Explain to the nurse that the patient is within his rights to refuse the procedure

e) Explain to the patient that he is in imminent danger of a fatal arrhythmia

Question 16: The fitting patient

You are the FY1 doctor on a general surgery firm. You are completing discharge summaries when you are bleeped by a nurse who informs you that one of your patients is having a seizure. Your SHO is on nights and your registrar and consultant are off-site at a clinic. There are no other doctors on the ward. You have never dealt with a fitting patient before.

Rank in order the following actions in response to this situation (1= Most appropriate; 5= Least appropriate)

a) Look up management of seizures on the internet

b) Go and assess the patient

c) Ask the senior nurse on the ward to assist you

d) Tell the nurse to instigate a management plan you think you remember from medical school

e) Bleep the Medical Registrar on-call

Question 17: A Distressed Family

During a busy weekend on-call, you are dealing with a sick patient. As you are taking an ABG to the analyser you bump into the father of one of your regular patients, he is visibly distressed. His son (your regular patient) was placed on the Liverpool Care Pathway the night before. The father tells you that he cannot take seeing his son suffer anymore and he is going to end his son's life to stop the suffering.

Rank in order the following actions in response to this situation *(1= Most appropriate; 5= Least appropriate)*

a) Apologise to the father that you haven't got time to talk as the ABG sample will spoil, then continue and call security

b) Explain to the father that you have to get the sample analysed and you are looking after a sick patient, but he should talk to one of the nurses on the ward

c) Ask one of the nurses to stay with the father while you take the ABG to be analysed, and contact your senior to explain the situation

d) Bleep a porter to analyse the ABG sample for you and listen to the father's immediate concerns

e) Inform the father that ending his son's life would be illegal and call the police

Question 18: A Consultant's Complaint

At the end of a foundation doctors' teaching session, one of the consultants spends five minutes complaining about the conduct of the junior doctors during on-calls. He says he continually receives complaints from the nursing staff on his ward that the doctors do not answer their bleeps, and that they do not go to review all the patients that they are called about. He tells the group that this is completely unacceptable behaviour and unprofessional. You know that on the previous weekend your colleague was on-call and escalated to the same consultant that they were not coping with the volume and pressure of ward jobs, and the consultant declined to offer any assistance.

Rank in order the following actions in response to this situation *(1 = Most appropriate; 5 = Least appropriate)*

a) Challenge the consultant and state that juniors on-call are understaffed and not supported adequately

b) Say nothing as some of your colleagues may not be working well

c) Record the number and nature of bleeps the next time you are on-call and present the results to the consultant

d) Make a formal complaint about the consultant's behaviour, including his refusal to offer and help when your colleague was on-call

e) Ask your Foundation Trainee representative to discuss the issues with the consultant and report back to the group

Question 19: Colleague calling in 'sick'

You think you overheard a fellow foundation year one doctor in the 'doctors' mess' boasting that he has called in sick on each of his weekend on-call duties in the last rotation, when in fact he had social plans.

Rank in order the following actions in response to this situation *(1= Most appropriate; 5= Least appropriate)*

a) Confront the doctor and ask him if what he claims is true

b) Confront the doctor and threaten to inform staffing unless he covers your next weekend on-call

c) Approach the doctor in private, in a non-confrontational manner, and discuss what he was saying

d) Report the doctor to the GMC

e) Say and do nothing

Question 20: In need of handwriting lessons

On your first day as a FY1 doctor, a nurse bleeps you during the ward round to ask you to come back to her ward as she cannot read your entry in the patient's notes and drug chart, and she needs to know the plan and what drugs to administer.

Rank in order the following actions in response to this situation (1= Most appropriate; 5= Least appropriate)

a) Ask the nurse to see if any of her colleagues can read the entry

b) Inform her of the medications and plan over the phone

c) Inform the nurse you are busy on a ward round and offer to come later

d) Ask the nurse to implement what she can from the plan for now, and that you will come later to clarify the rest

e) Apologise and excuse yourself from the ward round temporarily, then go and clarify the entry

Question 21: The sandwich

You are the medical house officer looking after a 98-year-old man with a history of stroke that has left him with difficulty swallowing and recurrent aspiration pneumonias. He has been admitted to your ward with aspiration pneumonia. After an MDT review today, he has been made nil-by-mouth and is currently being fed via a nasogastric tube. His daughter has asked to speak to you, and complains that you are starving her father by not allowing him to eat. She explains that her father has asked her for a sandwich and that she intends to feed him as his swallowing problem is unlikely to improve anyway.

Choose the **THREE most appropriate** *actions to take in this situation*

a) Explain to the patient that he must not eat the sandwich

b) Speak to the patient about his wishes

c) Warn the daughter that the sandwich could make her father more unwell

d) Discuss the patient's feeding issues with the dieticians and speech and language therapists

e) Listen to the daughter's concerns

f) Instruct the nurses to ensure that the patient does not eat the sandwich

g) Discuss the situation with your registrar

h) Observe the patient eating the sandwich, and make an assessment of his swallowing

Question 22: What are the results of my scan doctor?

You are a medical house officer nearing the end of your shift. You have been looking after a 68-year-old retired nurse, who was admitted with breathlessness and is very anxious and concerned regarding the underlying diagnosis. She undergoes a CT Pulmonary Angiogram scan. Before leaving for the evening your registrar informs you that the scan has confirmed a Pulmonary Embolism (PE) and is also highly suggestive of lung malignancy. He asks you to prescribe Low Molecular Weight Heparin and Warfarin for the PE. You return to the patient to re-assess her condition and prescribe the medication as instructed. As you are doing so she asks you for the result of her CT scan.

*Choose the **THREE** most appropriate actions to take in this situation*

a) Politely explain to her that as an FY1 you are not in a position to discuss the result of her scan

b) Offer the patient information about lung cancer specialist nurses

c) Explain that the scan has confirmed a PE and that you are waiting for the formal report

d) Explain that she has a PE that may have been caused by an underlying lung malignancy

e) Take the patient to a side room, and discuss the different lung cancer treatment options that are available

f) Explain that you are prescribing the appropriate medication to treat a PE

g) Call your consultant at home to talk to the patient (as the registrar has left)

h) Advise the patient that the team will discuss her results further in the morning

Question 23: Drop in saturations

You are the medical house officer and have been looking after a 76-year-old woman with a history of COPD who was admitted to your ward with breathlessness. She is diagnosed with a pulmonary embolism (PE) after undergoing a CT Pulmonary Angiogram scan. You go to the patient to prescribe low molecular weight heparin and warfarin. As you are doing so, you notice that she seems more breathless than usual and her oxygen saturation is now 90%, which is down from 92% earlier.

*Choose the **THREE** most appropriate next steps to take in this situation*

a) Ask the nurse to put out an arrest call immediately

b) Ask the patient whether she feels more breathless

c) Prescribe oxygen via reservoir mask at 15L per minute

d) Prescribe 28% oxygen via a fixed performance device (such as a venturi mask)

e) Perform an arterial blood gas

f) Bleep the on-call registrar to ask for assistance

g) Examine the patient's observations chart

h) Examine the patient's chest

Question 24: Locum here for a laugh

You are one of two FY1s on a busy urology firm. Your SHO has started maternity leave and a locum SHO has been appointed in her place. You find that within the first two weeks since the locum's appointment, you are working harder and there is less support available to you. The locum has been seen drinking tea in the mess on several occasions and at other times he is observing oesophagectomies in theatre.

*Choose the **THREE most appropriate** next steps to take in this situation*

a) Talk to your educational supervisor for advice

b) Ask your firm head to appoint another locum in his place

c) Bring the issue up in front of the firm at the next urology teaching session

d) Talk to your fellow F1 to see if she also feels that the locum has not been pulling his weight

e) Confront the locum and demand that he should be doing more on the ward

f) Talk to the locum over coffee and clarify the situation

g) Check at regular intervals to see that he is working and not in the mess

h) Seek advice from your defence union

Question 25: First time procedure

You are an FY1 on-call and have reviewed a patient with chronic liver disease secondary to Hepatitis C. She is unwell with fevers, loss of appetite and worsening abdominal distension. On examination she has gross tense ascites. On the ward round, your consultant asks you to aspirate a sample of the ascites to investigate for spontaneous bacterial peritonitis. You have never performed this procedure before and feel anxious about the possible complications of doing it.

*Choose the **THREE most appropriate** next steps to take in this situation*

a) Ask your fellow FY1 to perform the procedure as she has done it before

b) Ask your registrar to talk you through the steps of the procedure

c) Refuse to do the procedure as there is a risk of contracting hepatitis through needle stick injury

d) Cover the patient with antibiotics and leave the procedure for the post-take team tomorrow

e) Read up on how to do the procedure and perform it by yourself

f) Inform the consultant that you have not done the procedure before and do not feel confident

g) Refer the patient to the gastroenterologist to manage the situation

h) Discuss the situation with the patient

Question 26: Only the best doctor will do

You are doing a night on-call in your paediatric firm. A distressed three-year-old girl presents, accompanied by her father, with a dislocation of the radial head on the right elbow ('pulled elbow'), obtained when playing with her family. There are no suspicious circumstances and you wish to reduce the dislocation with a simple pronation-flexion technique that your registrar has explained to you. You have not done this reduction before and your registrar is busy seeing someone else. The anxious father tells you that he wants the 'most experienced doctor in the hospital' to perform it.

*Choose the **THREE most appropriate** next steps to take in this situation*

a) Offer to give the child pain killers

b) Discuss the father's concerns around the procedure

c) Tell the father that you have performed the procedure many times before and proceed

d) Tell the father that you are the only person available to perform the procedure

e) Advise the father to bring his daughter back in the morning when there will be more senior doctors available

f) Tell the father that you have to learn to do this reduction

g) Offer to see if there is a senior colleague available to supervise you

h) Offer to see if the registrar can perform the procedure later

Question 27: Caring for colleagues

You have a close colleague who you have noticed has been losing weight and looking more dishevelled. She admits to you that her mood is low and she occasionally hears a voice telling her to harm herself. She feels she is able to resist the voice and still focus on her work. She has already visited her GP once, before the voice began and was offered counselling, but is still on the waiting list. She is considering medication.

*Choose the **THREE** most appropriate next steps to take in this situation*

a) Inform her clinical supervisor that you are concerned about her

b) Perform a mental state examination on your colleague to assess whether she is fit to work

c) Advise her to go back to her GP

d) Inform her you do not think she is suitable to work and must take time off

e) Prescribe her anti depressants

f) Phone your registrar for advice

g) Inform the GMC of your concerns about the colleague

h) Discretely ask other colleagues who are working with her how they feel she is coping with her clinical workload

Question 28: Nightmare cannula

Pauline is a 67-year-old patient being treated for cholangitis with intravenous Tazocin. As her ERCP showed a stricture in the biliary tree, she requires an urgent CT scan with contrast to further investigate the lesion. The patient is extremely difficult to cannulate and her last cannula has come out. She has had four days of antibiotics, and has made good improvement; however, she is still due another three days of antibiotics to complete the course. The patient is adamant that she does not want to be cannulated; she demands the oral form of the medication (which is not available). She also says she'll have the CT scan at some other point in the future.

*Choose the **THREE** most appropriate next steps to take in this situation*

a) Contact the microbiology consultant to seek advice about alternative oral antibiotics

b) Emphasise the importance of completing the antibiotic course and the CT scan

c) Encourage her to let you have a go in cannulating her

d) Call your registrar who is doing an endoscopy list to come and talk to her

e) Arrange for an outpatient appointment of the CT scan

f) Phone her next of kin and request they persuade her to be cannulated

g) Come back in an hour and see if she has changed her mind

h) Get the CT scan done without contrast

Question 29: Disinterested Medical Student

You are teaching a group of final year students in outpatients' clinic during your gastroenterology rotation on behalf of your consultant. While one of them is conducting an interview with a patient invited for teaching purposes, you notice that a fellow student keeps texting during the consultation, fidgeting and later yawns. The patient makes reference to 'keeping people awake'. The first student has completed taking the history and usually what follows is that a second student starts examining the patient.

*Choose the **THREE most appropriate** next steps to take in this situation*

a) Send the student out of the consultation room before the examination begins

b) Call your consultant into the session and ask him to talk to the student

c) Confiscate the disruptive student's mobile phone till the end of the session

d) Ask your consultant for advice immediately after the patient and students have been dismissed

e) Ask the student to stay behind after the session and talk you through a gastroenterology history

f) Apologise to the patient

g) Ask the student to examine the patient in order to involve him in the session

h) Create an interval between history taking and examining and talk to the student

Question 30: A possible mishap

You are on-call when a nurse bleeps you about a medication that had been prescribed by the day team. She questions the prescription of Amoxicillin, which she feels has been prescribed at an inappropriate dose. You agree with the nurse and feel that the dose is high. The nurse asks whether to administer the prescribed dose.

*Choose the **THREE** most appropriate actions to take in this situation*

a) Tell the nurse you cannot change the dose as you did not prescribe it

b) Inform the patient about the possible mistake on the drug chart

c) Check the BNF and change the dose

d) Check the patient's clinical notes

e) Report the high dose to the on-call registrar

f) Discuss the high dose with the prescribing doctor the following day

g) Omit the evening dose and ask team to review the following day

h) Change the dose to the one the nurse is suggesting

Practice Paper
2
Answers

Question 1: Just hours before the operation begins

The correct answers for this question are:

E.D.B.C.A.

E - Inform the laboratory of the situation and ask them to consider ordering urgent platelets before the planned ERCP on the day

This option demonstrates that you have realised your mistake and that you are attempting to rectify the problem. There is no harm in using your initiative by attempting to get the platelets ordered in as urgent to ensure that the patient is not put at risk and that he can still go ahead with the procedure. The language used within this option, in particular 'inform' and 'consider', support this option as the first choice as it shows that you are exploring avenues in an honest and thoughtful manner, and utilising relevant members of the multi-disciplinary team. It can be argued that this option is futile as the procedure is elective and urgent platelets should be saved for acute cases, however, the wording leaves the choice in the technician's hands as they will have greater knowledge on platelet supplies. It would be best to attempt this course of action before informing the patient that the procedure has been delayed.

D - Bleep your registrar and inform him of the situation

It is important to inform senior members of the team about this, as their experience will help in such situations and they may suggest alternatives that you had not considered. However, it is also important that you take initiative and attempt to find solutions yourself initially before going to more senior members of staff, thus option E has been preferred above this.

B - Apologise to the patient for your mistake and explain that the ERCP will be delayed

The remaining options deal with how to break the news most effectively to the patient. While this is a vital step to take initially, the options above seek to find solutions to the problem before deciding that nothing can be done. It is important for a junior doctor to act with honesty and integrity. It is vital to maintain the trust between the doctor and patient. The following paragraph from the Good Medical Practice outlines the appropriate initial response within such a scenario.

'You must be open and honest with patients if things go wrong. If a patient under your care has suffered harm or distress, you should:

a put matters right (if that is possible)

b offer an apology

c explain fully and promptly what has happened and the likely short-term and long-term effects.'

(Good Medical Practice, paragraph 55).

C - Ask the nursing staff to go and speak to the patient regarding the mistake

This option is less desirable as it was you who made the mistake, thus you should take responsibility for your actions and apologise to the patient. This is vital for a healthy doctor-patient relationship. It is superior to option A however, as it still strives to explain the situation honestly to the patient, as is in keeping with GMC guidelines.

A - Explain to the patient that due to technical difficulties in the lab his ERCP has been delayed

It is not acceptable to deceive the patient, and to do so to cover your own mistake questions your probity. You must maintain an honest relationship with patients; not doing so will severely weaken the doctor-patient relationship and thus have a negative impact on patient care.

Question 2: Nutritional treatment over medications

This scenario deals with a number of issues, including good clinical care, consent and teamwork. The most appropriate order for the options would be:

B.D.A.E.C.

B - Discuss the complications of diabetes with her

This patient may not be aware of the impact of the suspected diagnosis, and hence it is your duty to explain to her how this may affect her health in order for her to make an informed decision about the options available to her.

D - Offer her a review by the diabetic team as an outpatient

The patient may not be averse to getting more specialist advice in clinic. Hence, this is a good option, especially as it means that the patient does not have to stay in hospital. Furthermore, the scenario states that she does not want to have medical intervention, this is something that can be explored in more details at the clinic. Ideally, a referral for the GP to review would be appropriate in this situation, however as the option is not available, the current course of action is relevant to take here. The GMC states that good clinical care includes *'refer a patient to another practitioner when this serves the patient's needs.' (Good Medical Practice, paragraph 15c).*

A - Respect her wishes and complete her discharge summary

Although discharging the patient without addressing the matter is not ideal, she cannot be forced to stay in hospital against her will. Her decision should be respected, as she cannot be treated without her consent. This applies as long as the patient has capacity to make decisions for herself. She should be made fully aware of the possible risks that discharge has. This is a preferred option to take than E as it complies with her strong wishes to leave hospital, which she has very clearly communicated to you.

E - Inform the patient that you think she should remain in hospital for routine monitoring as that would be in her best interests

This option is not appropriate as a patient has the right to discharge herself. The only types of cases where a patient can be kept against his/her will is if he/she lacks mental capacity or is deemed mentally ill and a risk to one's self and others. As there is no indication that the patient in the scenario fits any of these criteria, she is free to leave if she wishes.

C - Inform the patient of the importance of eating a healthy balanced diet, including meat, to ward off other diet-related conditions

While well intentioned, this is not a good approach to take by any means. It hinges upon imposing upon her beliefs and practice, and could in turn anger and upset the patient. Furthermore, the claim that meat is required 'to ward off other diet-related conditions' is not accurate.

Question 3: Nobody likes a bully

This scenario assesses the junior doctor's understanding of teamwork, problem solving and escalating appropriately. The GMC state that you must support colleagues who have difficulties; they also emphasise that you should challenge colleagues if they are treating others unfairly and without respect. (Good Medical Practice, paragraphs 25c and 59 respectively).

A.C.D.B.E.

A - Advise your colleague to talk to the registrar and explain how she feels

It is obvious that this is a very difficult course of action for the junior doctor to take due to her difficulties with the registrar. She obviously has some anxiety and is apprehensive to raise this issue.

Although it will require bravery, this would be the best course of action for your colleague to take for a few reasons. Firstly, it is the most direct and honest approach to take as opposed to escalating the issue to a consultant or above, which may cause distrust from the registrar, as she had not raised the problem with him before escalating, and could affect team dynamics further. There is a possibility that the SpR is not aware of his actions and no-one has raised the issue to him previously. Secondly, raising the issue with the registrar will yield two outcomes – either the situation will be resolved, or the registrar will dismiss your colleague's concerns in which case there will then be a better case to present to the consultant or another senior colleague. This will show an attempt at rectifying the situation before escalating, and will give the seniors more cause to be concerned if the registrar has already been approached. Thirdly, the scenario states that your colleague is 'worried' about raising the issue with the SpR; this does not express a complete objection to holding a discussion with him.

C - Tell your colleague to raise this issue with the consultant

This is a favourable option following option A, as it raises the issue to the correct person; the consultant is responsible for the effective running of the firm. He will most probably be the foundation doctor's clinical supervisor, responsible for her clinical development, and thus has an added responsibility to ensure effective resolution of this issue.

D - Ask her to email the foundation programme director

This is the next best option, as the foundation programme director has a high level of responsibility to ensure the efficient and smooth running of the different foundation programmes within their remit. Obviously, the first port of call after speaking to the registrar should be the team consultant, as explained above.

B - Suggest to your colleague that she takes some annual leave as it will help refresh her

This does not address the situation, and although it may temporarily relieve the pressure, will not help your colleague.

E - Tell her to persevere with him as it is not just her who finds him difficult and she is only there for three more months

This is the least favourable option. It is bad for patient care as a doctor working under such pressures is much more prone to making errors. It is also not conducive to effective team work. Finally, it is very unfair on your colleague and will not resolve the issue that other colleagues have also had with this registrar.

Question 4: Anxious relatives

This question assesses your ability to manage uncertainty and to adapt and respond to challenging situations. It provides you with an opportunity to show you are proactive and demonstrate initiative.
The most appropriate order would be:

D.E.B.C.A.

D - Speak to the family about their concerns

Patients' families can play an important part in delivering effective patient care. This option is first as it is vital to see what the family are specifically concerned about before going to assess the patient so that you have a better idea of what you are looking for. It is important to be receptive to the patient's family and explore their concerns, as the Good Medical Practice states *'You must be considerate to those close to the patient and be sensitive and responsive in giving them information and support.' (Paragraph 33),* all the while respecting patient confidentiality.

E - Return to the patient in order to reassess his symptoms

Once you have a better idea of what symptoms are concerning the family, it is your responsibility to investigate them. It may be that the patient was not able to fully express himself during the ward round or that his situation may have changed.

B - Contact the consultant

Although this is not a wrong action to take, it should by no means be the first thing you do. You need to demonstrate that you are proactive and able to solve challenging situations by yourself. By opting for this first, you show a lack of initiative that is contrary to the qualities a doctor should have. An effort should be made to resolve demanding situations before senior help is sought. It would be unfair to contact the consultant without first reassessing the situation for any potential changes since the ward round.

C - Discharge the patient as per the consultant's plan and ask him to re-attend if there are any concerns

This is dismissive of the family's concerns, especially as these concerns involve patient well being that the consultant may not have been aware of. This option is preferred to the nurse informing the family, however, because it appears the relatives are keen to speak to a doctor, and because this option at least provides re-assurance to 're-attend if there are any concerns', a safety-net which option A does not provide.

A - Ask the nurses to reassure the family that the consultant has reviewed the patient and he is fit for discharge

This would be the least advisable step to take, as primarily, the issue of patient safety has been raised which is being dismissed here, and secondly the family have requested to speak to a doctor. It demonstrates a lack of effective communication and an inability to take on responsibility.

Question 5: The referral bleep

This is an example of conflicting duties. The trainee may feel capable of taking referrals and want to demonstrate that he/she is taking increasing responsibility. The trainee may also want to support a colleague who has not been able to take a break all day. Indeed, patient safety maybe affected if the registrar is tired and not taking appropriate information on the seriousness of the referrals.

However, it is vital that a doctor recognises and works within their personal and professional limitations (Good Medical Practice, paragraph 14). It is very important for the trainee to be trusted to be safe, and not go beyond one's limits of competence.

The competencies tested in this scenario include commitment to professionalism, effective communication, problem solving, self-awareness and insight, patient focus, and working effectively as part of a team.

The correct answers for this question are:

C.D.E.B.A.

C - Decline to hold the bleep as you are not authorised and help them contact someone suitable (another surgical registrar)

This is the best response as it follows the guideline and offers the colleague support and a solution to the issue (Good Medical Practice, paragraph 35 – working with colleagues).

D - Decline to hold the bleep saying it's against the rules and you never get breaks

Thirty minutes is a long time for the registrar to be gone, and for that reason the bleep should not be left with an FY1 to deal with surgical referrals, some of which may be complicated and urgent. The reply may be communicated bluntly and in an impolite manner however this is a safer action to take than those below, with respect to patient care. The registrar should aim to look elsewhere before asking an FY1 to carry out such a duty.

E - Accept the bleep and inform everyone who bleeps that you cannot accept or decline referrals but will take the details

Choosing between options D and E is a difficult one. The scenario clearly shows that the registrar is in need of a deserved break following a long shift. It would therefore be reasonable to assist the registrar in taking a break. However, it would not be suitable for a junior doctor to hold the surgical registrar's bleep for 30 minutes, especially as there is no mention in the scenario of a contingent plan to get hold of him if you require in case of emergency. Calls can come from GPs around the area, from any ward in the hospital, and from A&E admissions, including trauma calls. Surgical patients can require immediate care at times, and surgical advice should be at hand for those seeking it. For these reasons D has been preferred over E. If the trainee makes it clear that he/she is not taking the referral, but merely taking a message, then option E would be more appropriate than the remaining options.

B - Reluctantly agree and inform your consultant of the registrar's irresponsible actions once the registrar returns

An FY1 should not hold this bleep for 30 minutes, especially without a strategy (as outlined in option E). This option does not describe such a strategy of handling referral bleeps, but rather states you are taking the bleep, and also is harsh towards the registrar. For this reason, option B is below E. It is preferred to option A, however, as it shows an attitude of discontent at holding the bleep rather than the dangerous mindset described in option A.

A - Agree and tell the registrar not to rush, you feel capable and want to help your colleague

This option demonstrates an unsafe attitude and therefore is the least preferred option. This is an example of dangerous behaviour and highlights what the guidelines regarding 'working within competencies' aim to eliminate.

Question 6: Second Opinion

This question tests your self-awareness and insight, and enables you to demonstrate an understanding of your own competencies.

The correct order is therefore:

C.D.B.A.E.

C - Inform the patient's family that you are not the patient's doctor and cannot alter the decision

While you should respect the family's right to a second opinion, it is important that you are clear with the family about your role. The New Doctor states *'F1 doctors must introduce themselves to patients.....ensuring that patients and colleagues understand their role, remit and limitations.' (Paragraph 9.b).* As an FY1 doctor, you are limited in that you are not authorised to make decisions on the resuscitation status of patients. In addition, as you are not a member of the team responsible for the patient's care, it would be inappropriate for such decisions to be made without prior discussion with the patient's team. In taking this action first, the family would understand that they should take up the issue with the relevant team in order to discuss the matter further, and therefore you are not dismissing the family's concerns by choosing this option first.

D - Explore the family's concerns with them

You may not be allowed to alter the DNAR status, but you are advised to be considerate and responsive to the patient's family as long as you are clear with them about your limitations. This option demonstrates your willingness to engage and communicate effectively, even if the family's primary objective cannot be fulfilled by you.

B - Contact the relevant team and inform them of the family's concerns

It is important to make the team aware of the family's concern. However, this is not one of the initial actions to take as it is more important to outline your limited position to the family from the start, as explained above.

A - Review the patient and discuss the suitability of the DNAR status

The following options would be inappropriate. It would be incorrect for you to review this patient, as the patient is not under your care. Furthermore, decisions on resuscitation should be made, ideally, by senior clinicians. This option demonstrates a lack of awareness of one's role and limitations.

E - Put a temporary hold on the DNAR status until you have had a discussion with the other team

This is a poor option as a drastically major decision about a patient who is under the care of another team has been taken independently. Like option A, this option also demonstrates a lack of awareness of one's own role and limitations. This is worse than option A as a hold is being put on the DNAR which is an inappropriate decision for an FY1 to make, especially without assessing the patient or discussing with the team first.

Question 7: Off home at five on the dot

This scenario raises a number of issues relating to working within a team. As outlined in Good Medical Practice, the junior doctor is expected to:

'When you are on duty you must be readily accessible to patients and colleagues seeking information, advice or support.' (paragraph 34)

'You must work collaboratively with colleagues, respecting their skills and contributions.' (paragraph 35)

The correct answers for this question are:

A.E.D.B.C.

A - Inform the registrar that you were unaware that there were jobs left and offer to stay behind and help to complete those jobs

In this example, a conciliatory approach with your senior would be the best way to maintain a positive working relationship. It is not uncommon for many senior professionals, rightly or wrongly, to expect the junior doctor to be the most proactive in the team in completing ward jobs. While it is normal for jobs to be allocated between team members, the reality is that all members of the team are responsible for ensuring that the work is completed and a high quality of patient is care is delivered. This immediate response of a willingness to stay behind and help complete the jobs is why this option is above E.

E - Apologise and speak to your SHOs about this issue and clarify the expectations the team has of one another

Speaking to your SHOs would be good practice as it may be that they are unhappy with the current state of affairs, and a simple conversation to clarify your position would benefit the team. To clarify what is expected of each other would only boost the team's efficiency in completing work on the ward and help to prevent future misunderstandings about what is expected from each team member.

D - Apologise and speak to your clinical supervisor about this incident

Speaking to ones clinical supervisor about issues that affect your working environment is very important. Such encounters contribute to a junior doctor's own learning and form part of self-reflection on practice, which extends both to patients and to other colleagues. In most cases, your clinical supervisor will be the consultant of the team. It would not be recommended for this to be your first action in such a situation, as speaking to those directly involved should be the priority. Furthermore, it may be that after completing points A and E, no further action is necessary.

B - Explain that you are not obliged to stay beyond 5pm as those are your contracted hours

This is an unsatisfactory response that would exacerbate a tense situation and potentially have detrimental effects to the workings of the team and consequently the care delivered to the patients under the team's care. While your claim is a correct one, the manner in which it is said within the current situation is inappropriate. It is more appropriate than option C because the content of your reasoning holds truth to it, whereas in option C, it is wrong to suggest that 'it is not your responsibility to do other people's jobs for them'. This goes against team working attributes required of an FY1.

C - Explain that you have completed the jobs assigned to you for the day and it is not your responsibility to do other people's jobs for them

This response is unlikely to help a tense situation where an obviously stressed senior is upset at the actions of their junior. While it may be the case that the jobs assigned to an individual are completed, it is part of good teamwork that efforts are made to help other colleagues complete their jobs.

Question 8: Third year wrestles with a cannula

The correct answers to this question are:

B.C.A.E.D.

B - Apologise to the patient for the failed attempts and insert the cannula yourself

The immediate focus in this scenario must be the patient's wellbeing and maintaining his trust in the medical team. The scenario mentions that the patient appears distressed, and thus this is the most favourable first step, as outlined in Good medical Practice paragraph 55.

C - Take the student aside and explain that he is not to attempt medical procedures without permission

The student should be told in clear terms that he has acted inappropriately and should be reminded of his limits on the ward. This should be done in a sensitive and supportive manner in order to maintain student motivation on the ward. However, the patient's wellbeing is always paramount and all learning experiences are secondary to this, and must never compromise the care a patient receives. As outlined in Good Medical Practice paragraph 40: *'You must make sure that all staff you manage have appropriate supervision.'* It would be more appropriate to inform the student first, before the nurse is involved, as there is a possibility that the nurse was unaware that the student was not given permission, therefore making the student most guilty in this scenario.

A - Inform the nurse in charge of the patient that students are not allowed to cannulate without permission and that in future the doctor should be told in the first instance if it appears that a student is preparing to perform one

In keeping with this theme, the nurse should be informed of the boundaries that medical students have in terms of procedures. This conversation should be done in private with the aim of maintaining the safety and wellbeing of all patients on the ward while, at the same time, not depriving medical students of important learning opportunities. It is best to inform the nurse in charge of the patient to prevent her from allowing any other students to attempt such procedures on the ward without permission, especially if she had been unaware of such regulations.

E - Inform the matron of this incident so that all staff members are made aware in order to prevent this happening in the future

The matron serves a very important role here in that she has unique access to all staff members and is a focal point in the management of the nursing team on the ward. Informing the matron of this incident will ensure all staff receive a timely reminder. This option does not directly involve the immediate persons involved, as do the previous options and therefore is placed as the penultimate answer.

D - Commend the student for his initiative and supervise him in attempting the cannula again

While it is important to reinforce the positive aspects of the student's action, that is to say the initiative in wanting to help the patient and the team, it is not an immediate priority here. The patient and family are currently distressed, and it would be unfair to allow the student to have another go. However, positive reinforcement is an essential aspect of effective teaching, especially for medical students attempting practical procedures that can take many attempts to gain competency in. This can further be expanded by a closer look at the Good Medical Practice guidelines on teaching and training:

'You should be prepared to contribute to teaching and training doctors and students.'

'You must be honest and objective when writing references, and when appraising or assessing the performance of colleagues, including locums and students.' (Paragraphs 39 and 41)

Question 9: ABG from the wrong patient!

The correct answers to this question are:

A.B.C.E.D.

A - Apologise to the patient you have taken the ABG from and explain it was an unnecessary procedure

It is possible that some team members may arrive late to a ward round. Post take rounds are often very busy and brisk, and arriving late can mean missing the review of a patient for whom you will later have to do jobs for.

The most pertinent action in this scenario is to firstly address the mistake of inflicting an invasive procedure on a patient incorrectly. This will involve an apology and an explanation of why this mistake occurred. Whilst unlikely, it may be that the patient wants to make a complaint. If this is the case, then he/she must be informed in full about how he/she can go about doing this according to local hospital policy.

Most patients will overlook mistakes as long as they feel their doctor is honest about the cause of the mistake. This is why probity is such a crucial aspect of good medical practice.

B - Take the ABG from the correct patient

The second step is to complete the task at hand and take the ABG from the correct patient. This supersedes the other options as it directly relates to patient care in the immediate term.

C - Fill out a clinical incident form and inform your senior team member of what has happened

It would then be good practice to complete a clinical incident form. This should be performed in conjunction with a discussion with your senior and/or the nurse in charge. These forms do not exist to isolate individual mistakes and embarrass doctors, rather they act as a timely reminder of mistakes that happen on the ward, especially in a high-pressure environment and help to ensure such mistakes are avoided in the future. This would be preferable to speaking to your clinical supervisor alone as it also adds a further benefit of completing a clinical incident form as well.

E - Discuss the incident with your clinical supervisor

This is good practice. Mistakes can be some of the most powerful stimulators to learning and increasing vigilance in clinical work. Reflecting on one's own practice, either alone or with your supervisor, is one of the many recommendations of the Good Medical Practice guidelines related to improving ones performance, *'You must take steps to monitor and improve the quality of your work.' (Paragraph 13).*

D - Keep the incident to yourself, as it has not caused any real harm to anyone

This is not the correct action to take. Whether an incident has caused harm or not should not be a factor when considering whether or not it should be flagged up as an incident. All clinical incidents should be discussed with senior colleagues and dealt with in the manner described above. This will help avoid such incidents from re-occurring and will also keep the members of the team updated on the care of their patients.

Question 10: A Stressed SHO

This is a scenario that many FY1 doctors will experience during the start of their careers. It tests a variety of skills – knowing one's limitations, working in a team and respecting your colleagues and of course, keeping in mind that the safety of your patients is paramount in every situation.

C.B.E.A.D.

C - Review the patient, and ensure that he/she is stable then bleep the SHO to confirm your plan

As a doctor, you are expected to be able to review patients' clinical needs. All junior doctors are apprehensive in the early weeks/months of their careers regarding how to manage acutely unwell patients. In this scenario, the best course of action to take is to review the patient as best as you can, formulate a plan and then contact your SHO if you are worried that you may have missed something. Often, histories given over the phone do not illustrate the full picture. Reading through the patients' notes carefully will give you a good idea of what is actually going on and provide clues as to the source of the acute illness. As stated in the GMC guidelines:

'You must provide a good standard of practice and care. If you assess, diagnose or treat patients, you must:

a adequately assess the patient's conditions, taking account of their history (including the symptoms and psychological, spiritual, social and cultural factors), their views and values; where necessary, examine the patient

b promptly provide or arrange suitable advice, investigations or treatment where necessary

c refer a patient to another practitioner when this serves the patient's needs.'

(Good Medical Practice, paragraph 15).

A key aspect of this scenario is appreciation of your limitations as a doctor. *'You must recognise and work within the limits of your competence.' (Good Medical practice, paragraph 14).* However, awareness of your limitations should not stop you from carrying out an expected duty i.e. reviewing a patient and deciding whether they require senior review.

B - Review the patient and then call the registrar and inform him of the situation and ask for advice

Contacting your registrar is a very viable and sensible option at this point, particularly having just reviewed a sick patient. It is reasonable to assume that he/she will also be very busy, but in the absence of your SHO being able to help you, it is logical to ask for the advice of the next senior colleague. It is important to stress, however, that one is encouraged to contact their registrar after reviewing the patient first, as all foundation year doctors are competent enough to complete a basic ABC assessment.

E - Offer to help the SHO with her current patients so that she can go and review this new patient

This option is a good way of letting your SHO know that you do not feel comfortable seeing the patient alone and also may provide relief to a stressful situation. It may be that the SHO has reviewed patients and created a list of jobs that she is now attempting to complete, and your help in this matter would allow her to review other acutely unwell patients. This is better than option A, as you are offering to help the SHO with her jobs rather than simply stating your discomfort at seeing the sick patient alone.

A - Tell your SHO you do not feel comfortable seeing this patient alone

As a doctor, you are expected to be able to clinically review a patient, and only after assessing them, should you be able to decide whether or not their needs go beyond your limits. However, this is favoured to option D, as you are being honest and seeking help from an appropriate medical senior.

D - Ask the nurses looking after the patient for advice

Often overlooked, experienced nurses are an excellent resource for a newly qualified doctor. However, it is important to stress that clinical decisions must come from a doctor, and particularly in this case where the patient sounds 'too complex for you to assess', one should not place reliance on nurses' advice without having first explored other courses of action (as in option E).

Question 11: Doctor in the family

The correct answers to this scenario are:

C.D.A.E.B.

This scenario raises the topic of patient confidentiality. The Good Medial Practice guidelines state:

'You must treat information about patients as confidential. This includes after a patient has died.' (Paragraph 50).

C - Inform the relative that despite being a qualified doctor, he has no right to look through patient notes in this hospital

The most pressing matter in this situation is to stop the relative from looking in the patients notes. He should then be clearly told that his status as a qualified doctor does not permit him to look through a patient's notes on the ward. An important caveat to this is mentioned in the GMC guidance:

'You must be considerate to those close to the patient and be sensitive and responsive in giving them information and support.' (Good Medical Practice, paragraph 33).

As such, you must make every effort to be firm yet polite in informing the relative of this error. Efforts should also be made to be respectful of his concerns and views regarding the patient as he is a relative, and is afforded the rights of all relatives in this setting.

D - Explain to the relative that it is the responsibility of the team in charge of the patient to decide what investigations are needed

He should then be told of the process by which investigations are ordered, that is to say, by the team in charge of the patient's care. Investigations cannot be ordered at the behest of any relative. Good Medical Practice states in paragraph 57:

'The investigations or treatment you provide or arrange must be based on the assessment you and the patient make of their needs and priorities, and on your clinical judgement about the likely effectiveness of the treatment options.'

Option D does not outline the issue of confidentiality as is done in option A, and therefore lies below it.

A - Inform the nurse in charge of the incident

The nurse in charge should be told about this incident as a matter of urgency. She will then be able to ensure such an incident is unlikely to occur again, and make other nursing staff aware of this incident. It may be that the patient's notes trolley was left unattended in the ward or this relative was not challenged as he stated that he was a doctor.

E - Document the encounter in the patient's notes

Once the immediate situation has been dealt with (as outlined in the above options), it is then important to document in the notes. This encounter must be clearly documented in the patient's notes because there has been a breach of confidentiality. The details of the encounter, as well as which other health professionals were informed, should also be clearly noted. This incident may be escalated if it is deemed that negligence on the part of ward staff contributed to this breach, and as such accurate documentation is vital to safeguard your role and that of other involved health professionals.

B - Ask your registrar to come down to the ward and speak to the relative

The immediate needs of the situation should be dealt with first before informing your registrar, particularly as this is a situation that can be addressed by a junior without the need for senior input initially. As with the vast majority of such encounters, however, it is good practice to inform your team of what has transpired so that they are aware of the situation.

Question 12: The cannula in a cardiac arrest

Foundation year doctors are part of the resuscitation team and their role is to assist in any way as assigned by the team leader. In an emergency situation, it is vital that the foundation year doctor is confident in their ability whilst recognising their limitations. Due to their size, large bore cannulae are generally harder to insert into veins.

This scenario addresses two main competencies: 'self-awareness and insight' and 'working effectively as part of the team'.

The Good Medical Practice states:

'You must offer help if emergencies arise in clinical settings or in the community, taking account of your own safety, your competence and the availability of other options for care.' (Paragraph 26).

Therefore the correct answers to this scenario would be:

C.A.B.D.E.

C - Voice your concerns to the team leader

In an emergency situation it is very important to know one's limitations and to be able to communicate this to the team. For this reason, informing the team leader is vital and this makes this option the most optimal answer.

A - Offer to take an arterial blood gas sample instead

If you do not feel confident in inserting a cannula and are more confident in taking an arterial blood gas, then this can be suggested to the team leader. In a cardiac arrest, an ABG would be required, so this is not an unreasonable suggestion to make. As you have been assigned to insert a cannula, you must communicate this to the team, so another member can attempt to gain access.

B - Insert a smaller sized cannula instead – after all access is access

The patient does not have any access currently and therefore it is more important to secure intravenous access. This option is more appropriate than option D because gaining access quickly is essential, and if a larger sized cannula is required it can be inserted at a later time. Likewise as mentioned above, you should communicate to the team leader what you are doing.

D - Attempt to insert a large bore cannula

If you do not have any other option, then you should attempt to insert a cannula despite not feeling confident. Waiting for the anaesthetist is not a reason to delay this attempt as is explained below.

E - Wait for the anaesthetist to insert a cannula after securing the airway

Waiting for the anaesthetist is an incorrect answer, apart from putting extra pressure and responsibility on the anaesthetist, one does not know how long it will take to secure the airway – resulting in precious time being wasted.

Question 13: The difficult arterial blood gas

Taking an arterial blood gas is a core procedure that a foundation year doctor must be able to perform. The case in the scenario is a common presentation to A&E.

The competencies highlighted in this scenario include commitment to professionalism, as a doctor must take responsibility of their actions, effective communication, as it is important to explain and update the patient about their management, and ensuring that the patient's care is always the primary focus.

The Good Medical Practice competencies being examined in this scenario are: Keeping your professional knowledge and skills up to date (paragraph 8), treating patients politely and considerately (paragraph 46) and listening to patients and responding to their concerns and preferences (paragraph 31).

It is important that the doctor apologises and explains to the patient that the sample isn't the correct one. The doctor should communicate with the patient as to whether he would mind a final attempt or would prefer someone else to have an attempt. In such cases, it is normally advised not to persist beyond three attempts.

Therefore the correct answers to this scenario would be:

A.B.E.D.C.

A - Apologise to the patient and ask if he would prefer someone else to try

As obtaining an arterial blood gas is a core procedure, it would be advised to first apologise and then discuss with the patient whether he would mind if the doctor had a final attempt. The patient may agree or he may wish someone else to try. The doctor should then respect the patient's wishes and communicate this to the rest of the team.

B - Call your senior house officer and ask her to try

If the senior house officer is not busy, then it is strongly advisable to ask her to assist you in obtaining the sample. It is advisable, in this circumstance, to escalate to the senior house officer before the registrar.

E - Ask the on-call registrar for further advice

If the senior house officer cannot help, then it would be advisable to escalate to the registrar. The medical registrar on-call is generally under a lot of pressure and should not be the first point of call in such a scenario.

D - Ask the surgical house officer on-call to attempt an ABG for you

The surgical house officer on-call is not part of your team and it is not appropriate to ask him/her to do this task. The surgical team have their own jobs to do and one should not burden them in this manner.

C - Leave it and await registrar review as the pH is stable

It is wrong and dangerous to assume that the patient is safe and stable if the pH is normal. In COPD patients the pO_2 will indicate if the patient is hypoxic and hence guide their oxygen requirement.

A venous sample also does not give the correct pCO_2 which is equally important in COPD patients and can affect their management.

Question 14: Coping with a heavy workload

It is widely known and appreciated that some rotations are busier than others. It is not necessarily due to a lack of competence or hard work that a junior doctor is working late or struggling, as described in the scenario. Being part of a team, it is important that the doctor is supported by his or her peers.

It is important that the doctor identifies that he/she is struggling and then analyses why he/she is not coping with the workload. It is important to communicate this to the rest of the team and to come up with a solution.

The main competencies that are being tested here are coping with pressure, organisation and planning, and knowing how to escalate such problems when they arise.

The correct answers to this scenario are:

B.A.E.D.C.

B - Reflect upon why you are taking too long

It is important, in such cases, to reflect on one's self. It is expected that a foundation year doctor should be able to manage and plan their work effectively. This involves prioritising and re-prioritising. If a doctor feels out of his/her depths, one should be able to identify this and seek appropriate help. Seniors do not expect their juniors to be constantly leaving late and to be working through lunch without having a break. This is not safe for the patients as mistakes can be made, and this pressure can adversely affect the doctor's health as well.

A - Discuss the situation with your consultant

It would be fair to initially speak to the registrar before escalating to the consultant. However, looking at the wording used within the choices, option A would be preferable than D, as the whole situation is being raised rather than specifically the teaching days.

E - Discuss with your educational supervisor, as you cannot see the situation changing

If the foundation year doctor feels that their education and training is being affected as a result, then it would be advisable to have a meeting with their educational supervisor and discuss strategies to improve their methods of coping under pressure, time management and organisation. This is preferred to asking your registrar to leave fifteen minutes earlier for teaching, as it deals with the situation as a whole rather than addressing the specific issue of arriving to teaching late.

D - Discuss with your registrar if you can leave at least fifteen minutes earlier on your teaching days

The registrar is responsible for leading the team when the consultant is not present and he/she should ensure that the team is coping with their workload. The bare minimum in this scenario would be to ensure that the doctor is able to attend their teaching on time. However, this option does not deal with the overtime into lunch and leaving work late, therefore is not as appropriate as the prior options.

C - Discuss with medical staffing and demand that a locum senior house officer is brought in

It would not be wrong to discuss matters with medical staffing in an attempt to see what options they can offer. However, the doctor would need to analyse his or her work performance first, and then escalate to the registrar and consultant who would then be best placed to discuss matters with staffing. To 'demand' a locum is an inappropriate first step and thus, this option has been ranked last.

Question 15: Fatal potassium levels

In order to understand this scenario, it is vital to have a grasp of the basic principles of the Mental Capacity Act 2005 and how it relates to everyday clinical practice. Although the patient has mild cognitive impairment, this does not preclude him from having capacity to take decisions about his care. The revised mental capacity act also makes it clear that a patient must be presumed to have capacity until proven otherwise (paragraph 1.2). It would therefore be unwise to take any action without first speaking with the patient and attempting to understand whether he is capable of making decisions for himself.

The correct responses are as follows:

E.C.B.D.A.

E - Explain to the patient that he is in imminent danger of a fatal arrhythmia

Explaining your own concerns to the patient is initially the most important step to take in this circumstance as his health is at an immediate risk. One should explain in a clear fashion what the problem is and how you plan to resolve it.

C - Listen to the patient's concerns about the procedure

Once the hyperkalaemic emergency is addressed, it would then be appropriate to listen to the patient's concerns about the treatment.

B - Assess the patient's capacity to understand the advantages and disadvantages of the procedure

It is reasonable, after first listening to the patient's concerns and explaining the potential consequences of his decision, to attempt to ascertain whether he has the capacity to make decisions for himself. The criteria for this are outlined in paragraph three of the mental capacity act. In summary you are presumed competent to be able to make decisions for yourself if you can:

a) understand the information relevant to the decision
b) retain that information
c) use or weigh that information as part of the process of making the decision
d) communicate the decision (whether by talking, using sign language or any other means)

D - Explain to the nurse that the patient is within his rights to refuse the procedure

Although the patient should be assumed to have capacity, this must not be taken for granted. You should attempt to speak with the patient yourself. It would also be extremely unwise not to discuss this situation with a senior colleague before coming to the conclusion that the patient is competent as the potential consequences are clearly very serious.

A - Explain to the patient that he cannot refuse treatment that is in his best interests

Informing the patient that he cannot refuse treatment can only be correct if he has been deemed to lack capacity. No evidence has been provided that this is the case and he must therefore be assumed to retain capacity. This option is the least appropriate.

Question 16: The fitting patient

There will be many times during foundation years that the trainee has to deal with a situation they are not familiar with. As with all situations, patient safety is paramount. Thus they must work up to but not beyond their competence, and know how and when to get help accordingly. Stabilising the patient, informing seniors and initiating appropriate investigations and management are expected from the junior doctor. Further optimisation can be done when senior support is available and/or the patient is stable. The correct ranking of options in this scenario is:

B.C.E.A.D.

B - Go and assess the patient

The most appropriate initial response will be to assess the situation; this will enable you to effectively prioritise your subsequent actions and seek appropriate assistance. An acutely unwell patient like this one should be assessed using an 'ABCDE' (Airways, Breathing, Circulation, Disability and Exposure) approach (it is expected that foundation year one doctors are able to carry out this assessment proficiently and instigate appropriate initial management).

C - Ask the senior nurse on the ward to assist you

The senior ward nurse will, in most instances, be readily available to help you deal with an unwell patient. As you work through your 'ABCDE' assessment, there are countless areas where the nurse's experience and assistance will be vital and thus this is a very good option. The reason this has been preferred to option E is because it addresses the immediate needs of the patient better and more effectively. The nurse will be on the ward and will be instantly available to assist with the unwell patient. The initial 'ABCDE' assessment is the first priority, and the nurse's assistance here will be vital.

E - Bleep the Medical Registrar on-call

As soon as the trainee feels that patient safety is at risk and they are reaching the limits of their abilities they must swiftly ask for help. This is reflected in both The New Doctor and the Good Medical Practice, which state:

'F1 doctors must demonstrate that they recognise personal and professional limits.' (The New Doctor, Paragraph 6).

'You must recognise and work within the limits of your competence'. (Good Medical Practice, Paragraph 14).

Thus option E is the next best option as the most appropriate person to call for assistance is the on-call medical registrar (as seizures are a medical problem).

'You must make good use of the resources available to you'
(Good Medical Practice, Paragraph 18).

A - Research management of seizures on the internet

As this is an acute situation, learning about the management while the patient is in immediate need of intervention is unwise and thus this option is ranked low.

D - Tell the nurse to instigate a management plan you think you remember from medical school

Patient safety is paramount and thus half remembered management plans are never appropriate. Pursuing this approach is unsafe and can be tantamount to patient neglect.

Question 17: A Distressed Family

This may seem like a far-fetched situation, however in hospital medicine, every once in a while, the junior doctor is faced with very difficult circumstances; this particular scenario replicates a real event. This scenario assesses the junior doctor's ability to cope under pressure, problem solve, decision making skills, and communicate effectively.

This is an extremely demanding situation both professionally and personally and certainly not one to be dealt with alone. There are conflicting commitments to different patients, relatives, staff and yourself. Any appropriate response will involve ensuring acute medical issues are being sorted, that the patients and staff are safe and that there is sufficient communication between the clinical and non-clinical staff.

The correct ranking of options in this scenario is:

C.D.A.E.B.

C - Ask one of the nurses to stay with the father while you take the ABG to be analysed, and contact your senior to explain the situation

The trainee must weigh the relative acute danger to both their patients and ensure both are seen to as quickly as possible. Option C deals with both the patients' immediate needs in an effective and succinct way. When the case is discussed with the senior, the trainee could offer to talk with the father as he is familiar with the case and request that someone else is found to look after the acutely unwell patient. If this is not possible, appropriate alternatives to address the issue can be reached. This option also shows a realisation of the limits of dealing effectively with both situations by one's self.

'You must recognise and work within the limits of your competence' (Good Medical Practice, Paragraph 14)

'You must offer help if emergencies arise in clinical settings or in the community, taking account of your own safety, your competence and the availability of other options of care.' (Good Medical Practice, paragraph 26).

D - Bleep a porter to analyse the ABG sample for you and listen to the father's immediate concerns

This option is similar to option C, however, in this option adequate use of the resources available is not being made. There are many other members of the on-call team whose help should be sought to address this situation.

A & E – (A) Apologise to the father that you haven't got time to talk as the ABG sample will spoil, then continue and call security & (E) Inform the father that ending his son's life would be illegal and call the police

The remaining options are all very poor as they neglect the very acute sensitivities of the scenario and poorly address the needs of one of the two patients. Options A and E both grossly misjudge the response to the father. The father is very distressed and emotional, he is in need of support and not confrontation. Option A has been preferred above option E as calling security will result in a more prompt response and thus help safeguard the son.

B - Explain to the father that you have to get the sample analysed and you are looking after a sick patient, but he should talk to one of the nurses on the ward

This is the least favourable for a number of reasons. The father has intense emotions and needs urgent attention. By not seeking help you are failing to comprehend the gravity of the situation that faces you, and you risk placing the son in danger. Also, simply explaining your other priorities and referring him on may make the father feel that you are neglecting/not valuing his needs.

Question 18: A Consultant's Complaint

This scenario assesses the junior doctor's ability to prioritise patient care, work effectively as part of a team, communicate effectively and demonstrate commitment to professionalism. Hospital medicine relies heavily on teamwork and good leadership, which require an atmosphere of support and trust. While it may be tempting to respond to anger with anger, one should consider the effectiveness and consequences of one's actions and work for the benefit of the patients and recognise the limits of one's abilities.

This situation is difficult because of the emotions involved and as the consultant does not seem to be consistent in his/her actions. The correct ranking of options in this scenario is:

E.C.A.D.B.

E - Ask your Foundation Trainee representative to discuss the issues with the consultant and report back to the group

A considered and constructive response is the most appropriate, thus this option is best. It is respectful and shows listening and taking into account the views of other healthcare professionals. An appropriate channel to address the issue is being utilised. The concerns can be expressed and discussed in a scenario where there are fewer emotions at play, and this will hopefully lead to an amicable solution being reached.

C - Record the number and nature of bleeps the next time you are on-call and present the results to the consultant

This option would provide some quantitative evidence to support your position and may provide a platform from which to work from. It may also involve working with others constructively to reach a solution. This option has been ranked second because it would be challenging to make this list while on-call, and thus option E was favoured as the most appropriate first step.

A - Challenge the consultant and state that juniors on-call are understaffed and not supported adequately

None of the remaining options are ideal, however, option A attempts to address the issue and has some potential to result in positive change as the issue is being raised (especially given that the other FY1s are also there and a discussion can result). It is to be noted that this potential is small, as being confrontational is very rarely constructive and is never professional and really should be avoided. In this case it may highlight to the consultant an issue he may not have considered but it is not the most appropriate way to make the point.

D - Make a formal complaint about the consultant's behaviour, including his refusal to offer and help when your colleague was on-call

Criteria 18 and 81 of The New Doctor highlight that there must be appropriate support and supervision for foundation doctors. Indeed Good Medical Practice applies to consultants as much as it does trainees and it states that all staff must be properly supervised and must be readily accessible to colleagues while on duty. However, going straight to a formal complaint without establishing the facts, attempting other avenues to address the issues or giving the consultant a chance to explain his position is inappropriate and does not show support or respect for your team members and certainly is not a good example of working together. Thus this has been ranked low.

B - Say nothing as some of your colleagues may not be working well

This option ignores the importance of the issue at hand. This is especially bad as it concerns patient safety and all members of staff have a responsibility to address matters that affect patient care.

'If patients are at risk because of inadequate premises, equipment or other resources, policies or systems, you should put the matter right if that is possible. You must raise your concern in line with our guidance and your workplace policy. You should also make a record of the steps you have taken.' (Good Medical Practice, paragraph 25b).

Question 19: Colleague calling in 'sick'

This case assesses the junior doctor's commitment to professionalism, working effectively as part of a team and effective communication. In this situation you are not part of the conversation; it is in a place of relative privacy and safety for doctors and you do not know the context.

It is not the foundation trainee's responsibility to judge, it is their responsibility to protect patients from colleagues' actions that may be deleterious and inform their seniors of justifiable concerns. Without exploring the situation further there is no basis or evidence to take to seniors or the GMC. The trainee must judge the situation in context.

The correct ranking of options in this scenario is:

C.A.E.D.B.

C - Approach the doctor in private, in a non-confrontational manner, and discuss what he was saying

This is the most appropriate, it demonstrates both respect for the colleague and acts towards protecting patients from risk of harm. The trainee should always act in a manner that justifies their patients' trust in them. The junior doctor must *'demonstrate respect for everyone they work with (including colleagues in medicine and other healthcare professions, allied health and social care workers and non-health professionals) whatever their professional qualifications, age, colour, culture, disability, ethnic or national origin, gender, lifestyle, marital or parental status, race, religion or beliefs, sex, sexual orientation, or social or economic status.' (The New Doctor, paragraph 10).*

A - Confront the doctor and ask him if what he claims is true

This is an appropriate action, namely exploring the issue, but undertaken in an inappropriate manner as you are confrontational. As such, it contradicts guidance on respect and team working.

E - Say and do nothing

The remaining options are all poor. However, option E has been ranked third due to the lack of information in the scenario. There may be a chance that you misheard, the context was different to what you thought or maybe the doctor was boasting, and may actually have been ill or may be joking. However, he may have called in sick when he was not and in that case the doctor's professionalism and conduct would therefore be seriously under question. Thus, this option is only ranked third as you try to clarify the situation in the two options above.

D - Report the doctor to the GMC

This is not appropriate based on the information given in the scenario. If after proper investigation it appears to be true then it will be appropriate. But the trainee must treat their colleagues fairly and with respect and support (Good Medical Practice, paragraph 36, The New Doctor 10b) and reporting people to the GMC based on overheard conversations is not indicated.

B - Confront the doctor and threaten to inform staffing unless he covers your next weekend on-call

This is a highly unprofessional approach as the colleague is being blackmailed into doing your on-call shift. It also implicitly condones the colleague's behaviour if indeed the colleague did miss the on-calls inappropriately.

Question 20: In need of handwriting lessons

The first day will always be stressful and no one wants to look slow. Ward rounds can be very fast and initially it can be hard to keep up. It is also vital to remember that patient safety is paramount, illegible notes and drug charts are a major problem for both patient safety and medico-legally. The New Doctor paragraph 6 articulates the necessity in keeping accurate and clear clinical records that can be understood by colleagues. The correct ranking of options in this scenario is:

B.C.E.A.D.

B - Inform her of the medications and plan over the phone

This is the best first step as it addresses the problem in a very effective and timely manner. Furthermore, it recognises that you are on a ward round and there are many other patients who also have needs that have to be addressed. Thus, as there is no indication in the scenario that there is an urgent need to treat the patient in question, it would be unwise to neglect the needs of many patients by leaving the ward round.

C - Inform the nurse you are busy on a ward round and offer to come later

This is similar to option B. However, option B supersedes it as a clarification is provided faster over the phone. It is positive that you are offering a solution to the problem.

E - Apologise and excuse yourself from the ward round temporarily, then go and clarify the entry

This is the third best option. Here you are admitting your mistake and acting to put it right. However, as has been explained above, it is inappropriate to leave the ward round to do this task and thus this option is below options B and C. Foundation doctors will continuously get requests to perform tasks, they must prioritise these and perform them in an organised manner.

A - Ask the nurse to see if any of her colleagues can read the entry

This option shows a degree of lateral thinking and trying to make the most of resources available. However, it is not good practice as there is a likelihood that your entries may be incorrectly read and the wrong plan implemented/drugs administered.

D - Ask the nurse to implement what she can from the plan for now, and that you will come later to clarify the rest

This is similar to option A. However, in this option you are asking the nurse to carry out whatever she can 'decipher' from your entry even after she has informed you that she is unable to read it. This can cause errors in the care provided and be detrimental to the patient's health.

Question 21: The sandwich

This question addresses issues relating to patient consent and autonomy, and highlights the importance of the Mental Capacity Act 2005 in everyday clinical practice. It also touches on relationships with patients' relatives. The Good Medical Practice states that *'You must be considerate to those close to the patient,*

and be sensitive in giving them information and support.'
(Paragraph 33).

The most appropriate responses are:

B.C.E.

B - Speak to the patient about his wishes

C - Warn the daughter that the sandwich could make her father more unwell

E - Listen to the daughter's concerns

B - The Good Medical Practice states that doctors must *'listen to patients, take account of their views, and respond honestly to their questions.' (Paragraph 31).* Thus, option B is very important in these types of situations.

C - This is important as the patient and his family need to make an informed decision based on understanding the potential consequences of the patient eating and re-aspirating. The risk to the patient of repeated aspirations is very high, and can potentially be fatal; this needs to be communicated clearly and consideratly.

E - The scenario clearly communicates the nature of the daughter's anxieties. It is important to demonstrate to the patient's daughter that you are listening to her, respecting her concerns and are devising management plans in liaison with the patient and his family. This option works well in synergy with option C.

D & H - The scenario clearly mentions that the patient has already been reviewed by the MDT today and that he is to be nil by mouth. Thus a new assessment is not indicated at the present time (D), furthermore you are not the correct person to carry out such an assessment (H).

A & F - Options A and F are both inappropriate without first speaking to the patient. The word 'must' makes option A unfavourable, as one should endeavour to involve the patient in decisions about his health (as is done in option B). Option A does not attempt to provide the patient a platform to express his thoughts and view, and is very authoritative. Option F is incorrect for similar reasons. It would also be important to establish whether the patient has full capacity in which case you must respect his wishes and decisions even if they appear unwise in a medical context (Mental Capacity Act 2005). All patients are assumed to have capacity, and this scenario does not indicate that the patient lacks capacity. If he did not have capacity, then it would be appropriate to act in his best interests, which may or may not include allowing him to eat.

It is important to appreciate that the daughter needs to be dealt with in a sensitive, non-confrontational manner. These options would serve to strain the relationship with the family.

G - This is a complex situation and therefore discussing the matter with your registrar would be wise at a later stage, however, the scenario requires you to deal with the issue at hand by speaking to the patient and his daughter.

It is likely that if you approach your registrar at this stage, he/she will advise you to go and speak to the patient and his daughter.

Question 22: What are the results of my scan doctor?

This question relates to providing patients with information about their care. Good Medical Practice states that you should 'share with patients, in a way that they can understand, the information they want or need to know about their condition...' (Paragraph 22). However, it is also important to work within the limits of your competence and recognise when others may be better equipped than you to perform a particular task. Where possible, one should avoid giving a diagnosis such as cancer on the basis of an unconfirmed report.

The most appropriate answers are:

C.F.H.

C - Explain that the scan has confirmed a PE and that you are waiting for the formal report

F - Explain that you are prescribing the appropriate medication to treat a PE

H - Advise the patient that the team will discuss her results further in the morning

C & F & H - These three options provide the patient with the current diagnosis which has been confirmed (the pulmonary embolism); they explain to the patient that the PE is being treated and state that further details will be discussed tomorrow. Information is not offered prematurely, nor is the (currently) confirmed diagnosis being withheld from the patient.

A - This answer is incorrect as it would not be unreasonable to discuss a diagnosis of PE and the rationale for treatment with the patient as an FY1. If required, it would also be reasonable to explain that the scan had revealed some abnormalities for which the cause was uncertain at this stage and that you are awaiting a formal report.

B & D & E - These options are inappropriate as the diagnosis of lung cancer has not been confirmed. Furthermore, it may not be appropriate for you to deliver this news to the patient, as she will almost certainly want further information regarding possible investigations, treatments and prognosis and so forth. Such management decisions will be made by your senior colleagues after detailed MDT discussions. You are said to be 'nearing the end of your shift' and therefore are not in an ideal position to delve into such a discussion at this time. Giving her incomplete information will add to her anxieties, and leave her upset and frustrated.

G - It would be inappropriate to contact your consultant in this scenario. The patient is stable and receiving the correct treatment. Furthermore, her CT scan is yet to be formally reported. There is little more that the consultant can add to her care at the current time.

Question 23: Drop in saturations

Clinical uncertainty is a part of everyday practice that you will be expected to manage frequently as an FY1. The Good Medical Practice states that providing good clinical care must *'adequately assess the patient's conditions, taking account of their history, (including the symptoms and psychological, spiritual, social and cultural factors), their views and values, and where necessary, examine the patient.' (Paragraph 15a).* On initial glance, this scenario does look quite clinical, however, what is actually being assessed is the approach and judgement one should apply when assessing patients.

The most appropriate initial actions to take are:

B.G.H.

B - Ask the patient whether she feels more breathless

G - Examine the patient's observations chart

H - Examine the patient's chest

B & H & G - Speaking with the patient about her symptoms will help you to clarify whether she has truly become more unwell (B). When assessing a patient, one should have a systematic approach, thus after the history the next step is examination (H). Following this, one can initiate investigations if indicated, starting with simple bed side tests and then going onto more complex investigations as required. Thus, looking at the observations chart will be the most logical step after examining the patient (G). It will quickly provide you with further information that will help you decide whether the patient has indeed deteriorated and if so, how severely.

C & D - The general steps that one needs to take are first to assess the patient by taking a relevant history, performing an appropriate examination and instigating the necessary investigations, and then deciding on a management plan. Thus, it is important that the patient is assessed prior to administering treatment and therefore both C and D are unnecessary at this stage. Furthermore, an oxygen saturation of 88-92% is acceptable for somebody with COPD according to the British Thoracic Society guidelines on oxygen prescription.

A & E & F - If the patient's respiratory function does deteriorate further, then options E and F may become necessary. If her observations are acutely worsening with severe hypotension and tachycardia for example, then option A may also become necessary. There is no indication in the scenario, however, that these steps are required at the present time. And even if one argued that options E and F were warranted from the information provided, they would not supersede options B, H and G.

Question 24: Locum here for a laugh

This scenario raises issues pertaining to teamwork and relationship with colleagues. As a junior, you should have senior support available to you. If the locum cover provided is not sufficient for the efficient running of the firm, then this needs to be addressed, as this could affect the quality of patient care.

The most appropriate responses are:

A.D.F.

A - Talk to your educational supervisor for advice

D - Talk to your fellow F1 to see if she also feels that the locum has not been pulling his weight

F - Talk to the locum over coffee and clarify the situation

D & F - Disputes may arise within firms and these need to be tackled in the appropriate way. Firstly, one should ascertain what the facts are, and hence asking your fellow F1 on the firm about her experiences with the locum would be useful. Furthermore, it is possible that the locum has not understood his role properly, and thus to talk to him in a non-confrontational, non-judgemental manner would be wise – perhaps he is having certain difficulties in his new job that could be easily addressed. Hence, options E and G are clearly not going to help alleviate difficulties in the firm.

A - It is always good to seek advice from your educational supervisor in times of difficulty as they may be able to help solve problems when other options have been exhausted. It is important to note that you are seeking 'advice' and not complaining.

C - This is wrong as it is not the correct forum for bringing up the issue and would embarrass the locum. Furthermore the facts have not been ascertained yet.

GMC guidance states:

'You must treat your colleagues fairly and with respect. You must not bully or harass them, or unfairly discriminate against them. You should challenge the behaviour of colleagues who do not meet this standard.' (GMC Leadership and management for all doctors, paragraph 7).

B - This is not an appropriate first step as your colleague should be given an opportunity to address the situation. It is unfair that this request be made without first attempting to rectify the situation using other means.

H - Contacting your defence union would not be the most appropriate initial response. The initial priority should be to explore the problem and try to use 'local systems' (e.g. your consultant) to address the issue. If that did not work, it would make the situation more challenging, and your defence body may be able to provide you with helpful advice on what steps to take. The GMC guidance states:

'If you have concerns that a colleague may not be fit to practice and may be putting patients at risk, you must ask for advice from a colleague, your defence body or us. If you are still concerned you must report this, in line with our guidance and your workplace policy, and make a record of the steps you have taken.' (Good Medical Practice, paragraph 25c).

Question 25: First time procedure

The correct options are:

A.B.F.

A - Ask your fellow FY1 to perform the procedure as she has done it before

B - Ask your registrar to talk you through the steps of the procedure

F - Inform the consultant that you have not done the procedure before and do not feel confident

B & F - The Good Medical Practice states you must *'recognise and work within the limits of your competence.'* (Paragraph 14). Hence being honest that you have not done the procedure is important. You will understandably be anxious in a situation like this, thus it is appropriate to involve your registrar.

This scenario provides a useful opportunity to learn a procedure – however, of the available options, there is no safe way for you to perform the procedure (under the supervision of a competent senior colleague). The closest option to this is option B, where you are learning about the procedure. It is always good practice to be supervised when performing procedures for the first time or when you are not comfortable in performing the procedure (thus option E is not favoured). The junior doctor must *'demonstrate that they recognise personal and professional limits, and ask for help from senior colleagues and other health and social care professionals when necessary'* (The New Doctor, paragraph 6). You should make yourself familiar with the risks of all procedures that you perform.

A - To ask the other FY1 to perform the task will lead to the aspirate being taken. Ideally, it would have been better for you to perform the procedure under direct supervision of your registrar or consultant, however, that option is not available. Options A, B and F work well together because you are informing your consultant that you are unable to do the procedure, while still informing him/her that your fellow FY1 will be able to get the job done, and at the same time learning from the registrar.

H - It is good practice to discuss the patient's care with the patient. However, in this situation, you are undecided about how you are going to deal with the situation to address your anxieties and lack of previous experience in performing the task. Thus, at the current time there is not much that you can really discuss with the patient.

D - This is an unwise option and is bad for patient care for numerous reasons. Firstly, the patient is started on antibiotics without a clear indication. Secondly, the ascitic sample acquired after a period of antibiotics would not be as valuable (in growing cultures) as a sample acquired prior to the administration of antibiotics. Thirdly, there is a long delay in acquiring the sample. Fourthly, if this option were undertaken, the junior doctor is not recognising their limitations and not asking for help when appropriate.

G - Eventual referral to gastroenterology may be appropriate, however, your consultant has reviewed the patient and has communicated a management plan, and this plan needs to be implemented. This option does not address any of the immediate needs of the situation.

C - To avoid doing a procedure as the patient has Hepatitis C is against GMC guidance.

'You must not deny treatment to patients because their medical condition may put you at risk. If a patient poses a risk to your health or safety, you should take all available steps to minimise the risk before providing treatment or making other suitable alternative arrangements for providing treatment.' (Good Medical Practice, paragraph 58).

Question 26: Only the best doctor will do

The scenario deals with good clinical care, honesty and integrity. According to the GMC, good clinical care should include referring *'a patient to another practitioner when this serves the patient's needs,'* and to *'recognise and work within the limits of your competence'* and *'take all possible steps to alleviate pain and distress whether or not a cure may be possible.'* (Good Medical Practice, paragraphs 15c, 14, and 16c respectively).

The correct options are:

A.B.G.

A - Offer to give the child pain killers

B - Discuss the father's concerns around the procedure

G - Offer to see if there is a senior colleague available to supervise you

A & B - It is important to understand the father's anxieties and to address his concerns. Although his request may seem unreasonable, good listening and communication could bring him round to the idea of a less experienced doctor performing the reduction. It is reasonable to want to learn the procedure, but not acceptable to be insensitive towards the patient's father.

The patient is the main priority and as she is in pain (and is likely to be caused discomfort by treatment you or the team will administer), analgesia is necessary. This will also help the father see you are a responsible doctor and may ease some of his concerns.

G - This is a very good option, as it will serve to reassure the father and also aid your learning needs, as you will be able to perform the procedure and receive feedback on performance. The scenario does state that your registrar is busy, however, your SHO may be available to supervise you.

C - This is dishonest and must not be done. Doctors must *'be honest in their relationships with patients (and their relatives and carers), professional colleagues and employers.' (The New Doctor, paragraph 11).*

D - This is not strictly correct, as there may be other members of staff more senior to yourself who may be available. In this sensitive situation where the father's concerns need to be listened to, taking an approach like that from the onset will only serve to sour the discourse further.

E - This is inappropriate because it will leave the child in distress and make poor use of resources, as the family will need to make another trip to A & E for the same problem that could have been addressed in the first presentation. Also, the same issues may potentially arise again.

F - It is true that as a trainee you have to get experience in performing procedures that you are unfamiliar with and have not done previously. In this context, expressing such an idea may communicate that you are placing your learning needs above the father's concerns. Expressing this thought will not help lead to an agreeable solution to the problem at hand, it is also unlikely to contribute towards building trust and rapport with the father.

H - This is a good option should the situation not resolve after you have explored the father's concerns. However, it is not an appropriate first response as the registrar has delegated this task to you, and there is no evidence to suggest that you do not feel competent in performing it. Obviously, if one feels unsure about the procedure they should readily ask for help and refer to another if needed. Furthermore, undertaking this option will mean that there will be a delay in providing the required treatment to the patient.

Question 27: Caring for colleagues

Your colleague is evidently running into difficulties if she is appearing dishevelled and losing weight, even though she has some insight into her problems. Given the circumstances, it is difficult to see how her condition would not affect her ability to work effectively as a doctor. Patient safety is the number one priority, and the GMC guidelines state:

'If you have concerns that a colleague may not be fit to practise and may be putting patients at risk, you must ask for advice from a colleague, your defence body or us. If you are still concerned you must report this, in line with our guidance and your workplace policy, and make a record of the steps you have taken.' (Good Medical Practice, paragraph 25c).

However, the situation still needs to be dealt with in a sensitive and constructive manner, you must *'support colleagues who have problems with their performance or health. But you must put patient safety first at all times' (Good Medical Practice, paragraph 43).*

Thus the correct options are:

A.C.D.

A - Inform her clinical supervisor that you are concerned about her

C - Advise her to go back to her GP

D - Inform her you do not think she is suitable to work and must take time off

A & D – The importance of patient safety in this scenario has been highlighted; thus you are duty bound to act on this concern, and notify an appropriate authority, in this case, your colleague's consultant. It may seem harsh to approach her consultant after she has confided in you, however the consequences of not doing so can be severe, both on your colleague and to her patients. The advice you offer her in option D, is very reasonable in light of the revelations she had made to you.

C – In the interest of her health and well-being, it is important that your colleague sees her GP urgently, especially as her care needs have significantly changed since her last visit, with the advent of auditory hallucinations.

B – This is an inappropriate option as you are not in a position to assess your colleague in this manner and pass a judgement on her suitability to work. In option D, you are stating your opinion that you feel that your colleague should take time off work, whereas here, you have taken it upon you self to make a decision about her health and ability to work. There is a dedicated occupational health team who should be involved, and are the responsible body that will make this decision.

E – The GMC advises against treating colleagues. Furthermore, it is inappropriate to commence treatment with the limited information provided by the scenario.

F - Your registrar may offer you some good advice, however, there are more obvious initial steps that you would be expected to make in a situation like this and thus it has not been selected as an initial response.

G - It is vital to support a colleague in such circumstances; obviously whilst supporting your colleague you must ensure patient care is not compromised. This option does not offer any support to the colleague; also, the best place for you to initially express your concerns would be to the colleague's seniors rather than the GMC. Thus option A is preferred.

H - There is enough information provided in the scenario that confirms the presence of a problem which needs addressing. This option does not act to address the pressing issues raised in this scenario.

Question 28: Nightmare cannula

This scenario assesses the junior doctor's understanding of consent, patient centered care, and respecting patients' wishes.

The correct options are:

A.B.C.

A - Contact the microbiology consultant to seek advice about alternative oral antibiotics

B - Emphasise the importance of completing the antibiotic course and the CT scan

C - Encourage her to let you have a go in cannulating her

A - This is an important step, the fact that the patient has rejected her IV medications should not mean the adoption of an attitude 'all or nothing care'. Suitable alternatives should be sought out, and the microbiologist is the best person to get advice from on this matter. Furthermore, seeking advice from microbiology does not mean you have given up on encouraging her to take the IV antibiotics.

B - This option is in the patient's medical interest and empowers her to make a well-informed decision.

C - Despite the fact she is 'adamant that she does not want to be cannulated', this should not deter you from your duty of advising patients on the best management options for their care. You may be able to arrive at a negotiated understanding where she allows you or a senior colleague to attempt the procedure.

D - Calling the registrar will not make a significant difference to the resolution of the situation, as there is not a lot more that the registrar can offer at this moment. You should do what you can to resolve the situation, and only escalate after that.

E - This is a poor option as many other avenues can be explored before the CT scan is booked as an outpatient investigation. Good practice necessitates that you attempt the other options and offer alternatives before resorting to delaying urgent investigations.

F - Contacting the patient's relatives and discussing matters pertaining to her health without the patient's consent has within it the potential to breach confidentiality, especially as the patient is assumed to have capacity. This may contribute towards the patient feeling frustrated, especially if you did not discuss the matter at hand in detail with her first.

G - This is a good option especially as the patient has been an inpatient for a few days, and giving her a little time to reflect on her decision may result in her accepting the advised treatment. However, before giving her an hour to consider, it would be more appropriate to first advise her on ideal management, particularly as urgent care is required, and give her the information to make a well informed decision.

H - The scenario states that the scan needs to be done with contrast, this is especially important as the structure may be malignant. Thus, doing a non-contrast scan will not help the matter as a contrast scan would be required to fully investigate the lesion. Even without this medical knowledge, an FY1 would not go against senior advice in booking scans, and would be required to run it by a senior first. It is not appropriate to expose a patient to radiation unless sure the scan is in the patient's best interest.

Question 29: Disinterested Medical Student

The correct options are:

E.F.H.

E - Ask the student to stay behind after the session and talk you through a gastroenterology history

F - Apologise to the patient

H - Create an interval between history taking and examining and talk to the student

E - This option has the potential to be a very effective response to this scenario. By asking the student to stay behind at the end of the session and expressing that you would like talk about history taking, a subtle warning is being delivered to the student. This should result in a change in behaviour as the student will realise that his behaviour has been noticed. It will also allow you to explore the matter in more detail after the session. Furthermore, it provides an avenue for teaching which the student has evidently missed during the session.

F - The patient has kindly given his time to participate in the session and has made it clear that he has noted the student's behaviour. It is important to ensure that the patient feels respected and valued; therefore a simple apology will be very important in realising this.

H - It is important to minimise the impact of his behaviour upon the rest of the session, so it would be appropriate to create an interval, perhaps using the excuse of a toilet break in order to minimise the impression of victimisation. This can create the opportunity to discretely take the student away from his colleagues and have a few brief words. A more detailed discussion can take place after the session, as has been selected in option E.

D & B - It is evident that the student's behaviour is inappropriate and impacting on the session, and that the rest of the session will be negatively impacted if the behaviour continues, thus it is better to attempt to rectify the negative behaviour at the earliest opportunity (thus option D has not been selected). It is therefore admirable to take charge of remedying it, without necessarily discussing the situation with your consultant first (thus option B has not been selected), but it may be considerate to make him aware of the situation, as he may be required to sign assessments on the student's performance, and will be encountering the patient again in the clinical setting.

C - This option is harsh, especially given that no prior warning has been given. It would be damaging to the student's self esteem.

Medical students are expected to demonstrate responsibility in their conduct and at the same time need to be treated with respect.

A - It is important that the student is aware of the impact of his behaviour, and the disrespect this reflects on both the patient and his colleagues. It is important to discuss his actions with him as there may be a reason for them, such as difficult social circumstances at home that may be diverting his attention. Therefore it would be inappropriate, as an initial response without a prior warning, to dismiss him, and also deprive him of a potentially valuable learning opportunity if he is able to remedy his behaviour.

B - You are the session leader and need to take responsibility of the situation, and exert initiative to resolve it. Calling the consultant into the session to address a relatively minor problem such is this is not appropriate.

G - Engaging the student in the rest of the session by asking him to examine the patient may ensure that the negative behaviour does not continue; however, this may be unfair on other students who have been participating well in the session as the 'disruptive student' is being more actively involved in the learning experience in preference to the other students.

Question 30: A possible mishap

It is not uncommon to come across possible mistakes made by your colleagues when working in hospital. The important thing here is how one responds to these situations. This question assesses your clinical decision-making, communication and teamwork skills.

The three most appropriate responses in this scenario are:

C.D.F.

C - Check the BNF and change the dose

D - Check the patient's clinical notes

F - Discuss the high dose with the prescribing doctor the following day

D - The patient's clinical notes are an important tool used to record the patient's progress and communicate with other professionals regarding actions taken in providing care. This option would be an appropriate choice as it would guide to why the antibiotic was prescribed, and if there is any obvious reason for using a different dose.

C - Your role is to make the care of your patient your primary concern. It would be very wise to consult the BNF to get clarifications about doses of drugs. This information, in combination with the information obtained in option D will help you make an informed judgement about the correct dose.

F - Discussion with the patient's regular team will serve to clarify the dose and amend it if it was incorrect. This clarification is in the patient's immediate interests, as if it is an incorrect dose, the patient may continue to receive that dose (e.g. if discharged with the incorrect dose).

E - In this scenario, calling your registrar should not be an initial response. The most effective thing for you to do would be to acquire as much information as you can and re-assess the situation. If you performed the actions outlined in options D and C; and still had uncertainties, then discussing the matter with your senior colleagues would be very appropriate.

A - This is incorrect as you can change the dose if there is a good indication to do so. If you are confronted with an error in a prescription, it is your responsibility to rectify this in the absence of the regular team.

B - Although it is important to be open and honest with patients, option B would not necessarily be the most appropriate step to take in this instance. This is especially the case as the medication has not yet been administered. If however, it was an incorrect dose and it was administered then *'you should...offer an apology'* and *'explain fully and promptly what has happened and the likely short-term and long-term effects.'* (*Good Medical Practice, paragraphs 55 b and c),* thus ensuring you do not undermine the patient's trust in the medical team.

G - This is inappropriate as omitting the dose may adversely affect the patient's wellbeing, it also demonstrates a lack of initiative in not finding the correct dose.

H - Nurses are a very good source of knowledge and support, however, it is the doctor's responsibility to ensure drugs are correctly prescribed, and hence it would be more preferable for you to check the BNF to ensure you are prescribing the correct dose.

Practice Paper

3

Questions

Question 1: Wedding day

You get engaged early in your Foundation Year One and quickly settle on a wedding date for the following April, which is eight months away. You immediately inform medical staffing and request annual leave for the relevant weekend and the following week. They tell you that there is no rota for that period yet, but that they will keep a note and there is no reason for there to be a problem. You contact staffing again early in the new year and there is still no rota, they tell you not to worry. A week before your wedding you receive a copy of the rota which shows that you are on-call on the weekend of your wedding and the following week. You immediately contact medical staffing and they tell you there is nothing they can do, it is your responsibility to organise swaps if you want the time off.

Rank in order *the following actions in response to this situation (1= Most appropriate; 5= Least appropriate)*

a) Remind medical staffing of your previous email correspondence and inform them that you will be taking the leave and ask them to help you find a swap

b) Accept the rota and rearrange your wedding at a week's notice

c) Accept the rota and try to arrange swaps at a weeks' notice

d) Inform your consultant

e) Make a formal complaint about medical staffing

Question 2: Reversing the Liverpool Care Pathway?

You are an FY1 on a respiratory ward. A 90-year-old patient who suffered from repeated episodes of severe pneumonia had been placed on the Liverpool Care Pathway (LCP – care pathway for dying patients to keep them as comfortable as possible) by the consultant as the patient was not expected to live for more than a couple of days. This decision was made with the family's approval. It has now been nine days since all curative treatment was stopped and the patient is still alive. The patient's daughter is very distressed and says she feels the decision to stop active treatment was incorrect, exclaiming that had it been correct the patient would have passed away by now. She demands that you restart all treatment.

Rank in order *the following actions in response to this situation (1= Most appropriate; 5= Least appropriate)*

a) Restart antibiotic treatment as the patient is still alive after nine days

b) Seek advice from the registrar from the other respiratory team (who is not involved in the patient's day-to-day care)

c) Tell the daughter that as the patient has been on the LCP for so many days, it is not in his best interest to stop it

d) Tell the daughter that the consultant who made the decision will be around in two days time and he is the most appropriate person to make a decision

e) Perform a thorough review of the patient and make a decision based on that

Question 3: You made the nurse cry

During a busy evening on-call, a nurse repeatedly calls you to re-write a drug chart. You still have three patients to review, all of whom are potentially quite unwell. You arrive on the ward to review your second unwell patient, and the nurse in question happens to be on that ward and exclaims that she had called you many times for the drug chart, which you still have not completed. In frustration, yóu use a few harsh words to emphasise how busy you are. The nurse starts crying.

Rank in order *the following actions in response to this situation (1= Most appropriate; 5= Least appropriate)*

a) Re-write the drug chart

b) Proceed to review your patient

c) Explain to the nurse again that the reason you could not complete the chart is because you are busy

d) Hand the task over to the night team

e) Ask the nurse to call the night team to re-write the chart

Question 4: Wrong dose and the patient has gone home

One of your patients has left the hospital half-an-hour ago after a successful endovascular aneurysm repair (EVAR) two days ago. The ward pharmacist rushes to you and points out that you had incorrectly prescribed a dose of Lactulose that is three times higher than it should be and that the incorrect dose had been administered for the last two days. The consultant reviewed the patient earlier today and deemed him medically fit for discharge.

Rank in order the following actions in response to this situation
(1= Most appropriate; 5= Least appropriate)

a) Ask the pharmacist about the adverse effects of the medication

b) Call the patient and ask him to come back

c) Phone the patient and ask him to miss the next three doses and inform him of the correct dose

d) Call your consultant to seek advice

e) Tell the pharmacist not to worry as you reviewed the patient a few hours ago and he was absolutely fine

Question 5: Racial abuse on the ward

You are the FY1 on-call, while you are re-writing a drug chart in a general medical ward, you hear racist abuse being aggressively hurled at one of the nurses by a middle aged, male patient. The other nurses rush to get your attention and ask for your assistance.

Rank in order the following actions in response to this situation (1= Most appropriate; 5= Least appropriate)

a) Do nothing, as you are quite busy and it is not your problem, there are also plenty of nurses there already

b) Tell them that there's nothing much you can do and advice them to call security right away

c) Confront the patient and tell him that this type of behavior is unacceptable

d) Tell the patient to leave the hospital as NHS staff are not to be treated in this manner

e) Prescribe some haloperidol to calm the patient down

Question 6: Family kept waiting

You are the only member of your team at your busy gastroenterology firm. You have had an extremely busy day as two of your patients required transfer to the Intensive Care Unit. You have another patient who wants you to discuss his complex medical needs with his family. You are aware that they have been waiting since midday and it is now 8.15pm. Your shift was scheduled to finish at 5pm.

Rank in order *the following actions in response to this situation (1= Most appropriate; 5= Least appropriate)*

a) Avoid the family on your way out as it is already very late and they may start talking to you

b) Sit down with the family and have a discussion with them

c) Explain to the family that you have been very busy with unwell patients and you can't talk to them today

d) Inform the family that you will speak to them tomorrow

e) Give the family a quick five minute summary and tell them you will address any concerns they have tomorrow

Question 7: Attending your prize award ceremony

You have been awarded a prestigious prize for which there is an award ceremony at 6pm at an external site. You are due to finish at 5pm; however, you get a bleep at 4.45pm informing you that a patient of yours is unwell. After assessing him you suspect a 'hospital acquired pneumonia' and you initiate further investigations. As the patient was already on antibiotics, you bleep your registrar, who is also the surgical registrar on-call, for further advice. As he is very busy in A&E, you have to wait 15 minutes for him to respond to your call. He asks you to prescribe new antibiotics and says he will come up to the ward after a further 20 minutes to review the patient with you. It is now 5.45pm and it will take you a further 50 minutes to reach your venue.

Rank in order *the following actions in response to this situation (1= Most appropriate; 5= Least appropriate)*

a) Call the on-call house officer and handover the patient to him/her

b) Go to the A&E department and explain your situation to the registrar

c) Call your registrar again and tell him that you need to leave

d) Try to find a different registrar to review the patient

e) Put the patient on the 'night handover' so he is seen by a doctor later, and leave

Question 8: Skiving off the post take round

You are a surgical house officer who has been called by surgical staffing to cover a colleague who has called in ill. Her team is 'post-taking' the thirty five new admissions from the previous day, and they are extremely busy. Due to this, you leave hospital 2 hours after your shift. The next day you hear that the colleague whose shift you covered was actually bride's maid at her cousin's wedding.

Rank in order *the following actions in response to this situation (1= Most appropriate; 5= Least appropriate)*

a) Ask the colleague to cover some of your on-calls to make up

b) Inform her registrar of what has happened

c) Express your feelings to her and come up with an appropriate solution

d) As this has only happened once, do nothing

e) Inform your consultant of the situation and suggest that your colleague should be asked to help your team during your next post take ward round

Question 9: Can't get work off my mind

You have completed your evening on-call and have returned home. Once home, you think back to Mr. Nicholas whom you catheterised a few hours ago. You are not 100% sure whether you retracted his foreskin after completing the procedure.

Rank in order the following actions in response to this situation (1= Most appropriate; 5= Least appropriate)

a) Check that the patient is well and there are no complications with the catheter first thing next morning

b) Phone the night SHO covering the wards and ask her to check that the catheter is okay

c) Phone the ward nurses from home and ask them to check that the catheter is okay

d) Go back to hospital to check on the patient, as you were the one who placed the catheter in

e) Call the patient's team the next day to ensure that the patient is well and does not have any problems

Question 10: Too many referrals!

You have just started your new job as a surgical FY1. During your very first on-call, the SHO who is on-call with you is suddenly called down to theatres. The locum SpR is not answering his bleep. All the A&E referrals, for patients to be taken under the care of the surgical team, start coming to you and you become extremely stressed. It has been two hours now and both the SHO and the SpR are still unavailable.

Rank in order *the following actions in response to this situation (1= Most appropriate; 5= Least appropriate)*

a) Turn your bleep off for half an hour as it is stressing you out

b) Reject all incoming referrals explaining the situation to the caller

c) Call the consultant surgeon at his home phone, through the switchboard, and ask him to resolve the problem

d) Discuss the situation with the A&E registrar and ask him to deal with the surgical patients for the time being

e) Accept the referrals explaining that you are the only team member around for the time being

Question 11: Just trying to relax with your flatmates

You come home after a good day at work. While playing some computer games with flatmates, you get a call from a patient's relative on your mobile phone. The relative has some important questions to ask about his father's health, and he explains that he obtained your number from one of the other junior doctors on the ward.

Rank in order the following actions in response to this situation (1= Most appropriate; 5= Least appropriate)

a) Tell the relative it is your private line and you won't be speaking to him now, and that your colleague made a big mistake in giving him your number

b) Explain to the relative that the earliest you can discuss the patient's care is tomorrow morning

c) Have a quick discussion with the relative and say that you can provide more details tomorrow

d) Advise the relative that the nurse taking care of the patient would be the best point of call at this time

e) Ask the relative to hand the phone over to the colleague who gave them your number and reprimand her for giving out your number without asking you first

Question 12: Final year student lets slip

You are attending to a 70-year-old patient who has a very suspicious looking chest x ray, that may show a tumour. Your team has arranged a CT scan to better visualise this lesion. The patient is unaware of this suspicion, as nothing has been confirmed yet. A final year medical student, who has performed a respiratory exam on the patient, tells the patient that she may have cancer based on the entries in the notes. The patient becomes very distressed and asks you if she has cancer.

Rank in order the following actions in response to this situation (1= Most appropriate; 5= Least appropriate)

a) Advise the medical student that he should not have made the remark

b) Reassure the patient telling her that she'll be fine

c) Phone your registrar and ask her to come up from clinic to update the patient on the current situation

d) Tell the patient that the medical team will answer her questions after the CT scan is done

e) Inform the patient that the consultant is doing a ward round tomorrow and she will be able to answer any questions that the patient has

Question 13: Colleague gone AWOL

You have completed your 12 hour surgical on-call shift and are going to the handover meeting. The 20-minute handover meeting has now ended; however, there is no sign of the locum night SHO. The night registrar asks you to hold the SHO bleep and take referrals while he liaises with the site manager to 'sort something out'.

Rank in order *the following actions in response to this situation (1= Most appropriate; 5= Least appropriate)*

a) Hold the bleep and wait for the registrar to address the issue, or for the locum to arrive

b) Explain to the registrar that you have just completed a long shift and can't hold onto the bleep

c) Tell the registrar that you'll hold the bleep for a further half an hour

d) Suggest that the register would be able to cope with the SHO bleep for a little while as the last few hours have been very quiet

e) Offer to cover the night shift on the condition that you are paid locum rates for your services

Question 14: Patient fed up and wants to go home

You have a long-standing patient who has multiple medical problems including a newly diagnosed colon cancer. The patient is still unaware of the diagnosis because you were waiting for the consultant to break the news in his ward round at the end of the week. The patient is adamant that she wishes to return home as she has been in hospital for 'six weeks now' and is now 'fed up!'

Rank in order the following actions in response to this situation *(1= Most appropriate; 5= Least appropriate)*

a) Break the news to the patient and tell her that she needs to stay for some further tests

b) Explain to the patient that her latest investigations have shown abnormal results and the consultant will confirm these findings with her

c) Offer her a 'discharge against medical advice form'

d) Call a family member and ask them to persuade the patient to stay, explaining to them the latest diagnosis

e) Find out if your consultant or registrar can break the news any sooner

Question 15: FY2 intruding

A 93-year-old patient is admitted under your team. This patient's grandson happens to have a close friend who is a surgical FY2 in the hospital. The FY2 regularly comes up to your ward to ask you about the patient's progress, he also reads the notes at each visit and relays his interpretations of the different entries to the patient's relatives. You become slightly frustrated because a person who is not a member of the team is giving medical updates to the relatives.

Rank in order the following actions in response to this situation *(1= Most appropriate; 5= Least appropriate)*

a) Speak to the FY2 in question and request he stops communicating each entry in the notes to the relatives

b) Discuss the problem with your registrar and ask him to speak to the FY2

c) Explain politely to the patient's relatives that the medical team are the best point of call for any enquiries they may have

d) Let the FY2 continue as he is, as it is not harming the patient in any way

e) Contact the FY2's registrar and request that she ask him to stop coming up the ward

Question 16: Reprimanded for minor error

The FY2 on your team has just been told off by the registrar for a relatively minor error. This has unfortunately happened in front of the patient as well as other members of the Multidisciplinary Team (MDT). The FY2 is obviously very distressed by this.

Rank in order the following actions in response to this situation (1= Most appropriate; 5= Least appropriate)

a) Rectify the minor error

b) Reassure the FY2 and tell him that it was actually quite a minor thing and the registrar over reacted

c) Talk to your registrar explaining that it would have been better to give the criticism in private

d) Inform your consultant of what has happened

e) Reassure the patient and tell her not to worry

Question 17: A kind gesture

An elderly patient is preparing to leave the ward after being discharged. He is pleased with the way you treated him, and he hands you a £50 note on his way out, insisting you take it.

Rank in order the following actions in response to this situation (1= Most appropriate; 5= Least appropriate)

a) Thank him for his generosity and accept his gift

b) Refuse the money and state it is against rules

c) Tell him it would be better to add it to the ward fund instead

d) Tell him that £50 is too much and if anything to give you half of that

e) Tell him a thank-you card would do

Question 18: All I'm asking for is to go to theatres

You are the house officer on a very busy general surgical ward. Your SHO regularly goes into theatres after ward rounds leaving the ward jobs for you to complete. You are also very keen to get some theatre experience, however, you do not seem to be able to get the opportunity.

Rank in order the following actions in response to this situation (1= Most appropriate; 5= Least appropriate

a) Voice your concerns to your consultant that there is an unfair distribution of the ward duties

b) Ask your educational supervisor to talk to the SHO

c) Sit down with the SHO and explain how you feel

d) Ask the registrar to discuss the situation with the SHO

e) Go to theatres for a few hours, directly after the ward round and then return to do your jobs

Question 19: Parents will 'have a go'

You clerk in a 16-year-old patient who has been brought to A&E from school, presenting with diabetic ketoacidosis. The patient admits to poor adherence to his insulin, explaining that he feels embarrassed to inject himself when he is at school with his friends. He tells you not to discuss this with his parents when they arrive as they'll 'have a go at him'.

Rank in order the following actions in response to this situation (1= Most appropriate; 5= Least appropriate)

a) Accept his wishes and tell him you won't mention it to his parents

b) Respect the patient's wishes, but explain that you feel it is in his best interest to inform his parents

c) Inform his parents as they have parental responsibility over him

d) Phone the head teacher of the school and explain the situation

e) Call the diabetic nurse to come and speak to the patient

Question 20: Squeamish patient & the blood cultures

You are working on a busy surgical ward and have a patient that you need to take blood cultures from as he has developed a high fever from a pneumonia. The patient is very reluctant to be bled, as he has had bad experiences with doctors being unable to bleed his very thin veins. You convince him of the importance of the test, and manage to successfully draw the blood after two failed attempts. Just as you are about to drop the sample to the laboratory, you realise your sample was NOT acquired in a sterile manner and thus may be contaminated.

Rank in order *the following actions in response to this situation (1= Most appropriate; 5= Least appropriate)*

a) Ask a nurse to return and take bloods again

b) Return and apologise to the patient for your mistake and offer to take blood again

c) Send the bloods off anyway as the laboratory should be able to distinguish between pneumonia-causing pathogens and anything else that may have been caught from the patient's bedside

d) Bleep your registrar and inform him of the situation

e) Inform the laboratory of the situation and ask them to consider the non-sterile conditions when analysing the bottles you are due to send

Question 21: Dealing with death

You find yourself on the ward without an SHO or registrar as they are on-call and your consultant is in clinic. A patient has a cardiac arrest on the ward and a crash call is put out, but unfortunately the resuscitation was unsuccessful. The crash team leaves for another call. Once you certify the patient's death, the nurse informs you that the family are on their way up and are not aware of the patient's death.

*Choose the **THREE** most appropriate actions to take in this situation*

a) Inform the nurse that you are a junior doctor and have been advised not to break such news

b) Contact your consultant to update him

c) Ask the senior nurse to take the family to a quiet room

d) Take the family to a quiet room and say that you will try and contact a senior doctor to come and update them

e) Inform the family of the death

f) Inform the Human Resources department about the lack of doctors on the ward

g) Ask the health care assistant to ensure the patient's body is in a dignified state

h) Apologise to the family that there are no senior doctors on the ward

Question 22: Lazy colleague

While working on a busy surgical firm you become increasingly stressed at your colleague who does not put in the same effort as yourself. He repeatedly arrives late in the morning leaving the patient list preparation to you and leaves no later than 5pm, claiming it's the on-call team's duty to work after hours, not his.

*Choose the **THREE** most **appropriate** actions to take in this situation*

a) Write an email to the Foundation Programme Director

b) Inform your registrar of the situation and ask him to kindly advise your colleague

c) Speak to your consultant about the stress you are undergoing due to the situation

d) Explore reasons for your colleague's attitude and offer support if required

e) Avoid raising the issue with your colleague directly in order to maintain your working relationship

f) Advise your colleague to attend work on time

g) Arrange a meeting with the registrar and your colleague to discuss the issue

h) Tell your colleague that his conduct is unfair and stressing you out

Question 23: Heartbroken

You are one of four FY1s on-call over the busy bank holiday weekend. One of your FY1 colleagues, who should have been present at handover, is not there. You presume she is running late and continue with your jobs. At midday you receive a text from the FY1 who was missing in the morning handover meeting saying she won't be turning up as she has just broken up with her boyfriend and is not in the right state of mind to come in to work.

*Choose the **THREE most appropriate** actions to take in this situation*

a) Inform the registrar on-call

b) Call your colleague and explain that it is a bank holiday weekend and therefore extremely busy, and she should come in straight away

c) Continue with your jobs and attempt to do as much as you can

d) Speak to your colleague's clinical supervisor

e) Call your colleague and try to comfort her

f) Advise her to take a few days annual leave if she thinks it will affect her work

g) Suggest she calls her seniors and lets them know of the situation

h) Discuss the staffing challenges with the other juniors on-call

Question 24: 'It's a free country'

Your patient is awaiting a pacemaker following a collapse caused by a life threatening arrhythmia. He ignores medical advice and keeps leaving the ward to go outside for a cigarette even after being told by the ward nurses that it is vital he stays by his bedside, on the cardiac monitor.

*Choose the **THREE most appropriate** actions to take in this situation*

a) Ask him to sign a document saying he understands the risks associated with leaving the ward

b) Emphasise the risks involved if he doesn't stay connected to the monitor

c) Call security to ensure the patient stays in his bed

d) Ask one of the nurses to stay with him and ensure he doesn't leave

e) Call his next of kin and inform them of the whole situation so they can persuade him not to leave

f) Ask one of the nurses to go out with him when he goes to smoke his cigarette

g) Respect the patient's decision. Let him come and go as he pleases

h) Inform the patient that if he is not willing to adhere to the medical advice being offered he should self discharge

Question 25: You lose your cool at the nurse

You are working through your long list of jobs on your chronically short staffed Gastroenterology firm when, towards the end of the day, a nurse calls to inform you that one of your patients has a small rash on her bottom. The patient is very stable and is mobile, thus you are not too concerned by this rash. The nurse, however, demands that you come to see the patient today. Due to your workload, you do not manage to see the patient that day. The next day, the same nurse calls you accusing you of neglect and poor patient care, and out of frustration, you put the phone down on her. When you see her on the ward she has completed an 'Incident Report' against you for not reviewing the patient yesterday and is threatening to call your consultant.

Choose the **THREE most appropriate** *actions to take in this situation*

a) Apologise to the nurse for putting the phone down on her

b) Hold your ground about not reviewing the rash yesterday as you had other priorities

c) Tell the nurse that her behaviour is intimidating and you will report her to the ward sister

d) Phone your consultant before the nurse gets through to him to explain the situation

e) Discuss the case with your registrar and ask for his support

f) Go and explain the situation to the patient, who you know will support you

g) Try to gain the support of an FY2 on the ward and ask her to intervene on your behalf

h) Go and perform a detailed review of the patient and document your findings

Question 26: Doctor, She's turned red

You are the surgical house officer on-call, and you have been asked to review a patient who is in some pain post operatively. You quickly change the regular Paracetamol to Co-codamol and then attend to another patient who is quite unwell. The nurse taking care of the first patient calls you a few hours later informing you that the patient was actually allergic to Codeine, and has developed a red rash on her chest as well as both arms. You rush back to the patient, stop the Co-codamol, and review the patient, who is well other than the rash.

*Choose the **THREE** most appropriate actions to take in this situation*

a) Reassure the patient that she will be fine

b) Commence management for acute anaphylaxis

c) Prescribe Tramadol for pain control

d) Prescribe Morphine for pain relief

e) Phone the on-call medical registrar and get his opinion

f) Apologise to the patient for the mistake

g) Place the patient on evening handover to ensure that she does not deteriorate

h) Refer the patient for allergy testing to find out what else she is allergic to

Question 27: The rush to discharge

You are the on-call house officer in a busy medical assessment unit. You are informed that a patient who is currently being managed for pyelonephritis, has spiked a temperature of 39.2 degrees Celsius. At the same time the nurse informs you that she is urgently waiting for a discharge summary for a patient who is medically fit to go home but has a blood pressure of 190/80 mmHg – she is known to have hypertension, but has refused her regular medications today.

The nurse is absolutely adamant that the discharge summary should take priority, as she needs the bed. She is aware that your on-call shift ends in 15 minutes and that the discharge summary has not yet been started.

*Choose the **THREE most appropriate** actions to take in this situation*

a) Explain to the nurse that you won't be able to do her discharge summary as the other patient is more of a priority

b) Ensure that the patient with pyelonephritis is on antibiotics and fluids and then proceed to the discharge summary

c) Miss the evening handover meeting and assess the patient with a fever and then do the discharge summary

d) Seek advice from a senior as to what to do

e) Complete the discharge summary so the patient can go home and the bed can be made free

f) Ask the SHO on-call to help you

g) Complain to the ward sister about the nurse's confrontational approach

h) Handover both patients to the night team

Question 28: No harm in exaggerating?

During a ward round, your consultant becomes annoyed that Mr. Jones has yet to have a CT chest scan. He informs you that he expects the scan to be done today without fail. While filling out the request form, your SHO tells you to exaggerate the patient's condition. She also asks you to write down extra details that are untrue, in order to ensure the scan is done as a priority.

Choose the **THREE** *most appropriate actions to take in this situation*

a) Fill out the form and exaggerate only certain clinical details to ensure the CT scan is done without delay, as this is in the patient's best interests

b) Refuse to write details that are untrue and say that you will speak directly to the radiologist and try to persuade him/her to perform the scan today

c) Tell your SHO you do not feel comfortable writing details that are not true on the form

d) Ask your registrar what the best course of action to take is

e) Fill out the form exactly as the SHO has suggested because she has more experience in ensuring scans get done, and it is in the patient's best interests to have the scan done today

f) Speak directly to your consultant about how to get the scan done today

g) Leave the form for the SHO to fill out

h) Fill out the form as suggested by your SHO on this occasion, but make sure in future that scans are requested early to prevent this from happening again

Question 29: Jehovah's Witness and blood transfusions

You are the medical house officer on-call, you clerk a patient who has presented with a query GI bleed. The patient's haemoglobin comes back as 7.3 g/dL and she requires a blood transfusion. The patient is a Jehovah's Witness and refuses any blood products.

*Choose the **THREE** most appropriate actions to take in this situation*

a) Accept the patient's wishes and document it in the notes

b) Persuade the patient to have the transfusion, explaining that otherwise she risks of death

c) Cross match a few units of blood in case the patient deteriorates further and becomes unconscious, in which case you would act in her best interest and administer the blood

d) Do a 'group and save' in case the patient changes her mind

e) Refer the patient for palliative care to keep her comfortable as she is refusing life saving treatment and thus has a poor prognosis

f) Offer to contact the patient's partner and hold a family discussion

g) Refer the case to the medical registrar and ask him to help deal with the situation

h) Ask the chaplain to try to convince the patient to have the blood transfusion

Question 30: Compulsory FY1 teaching dilemma

You are a medical house officer on a busy ward, as your SHO is on night shifts, it is only you and your registrar on the ward. There are no acutely unwell patients and it is almost time for your weekly 'compulsory FY1 teaching session'. You inform your registrar that you'll be away for an hour due to this, however, he demands that you stay and miss the teaching, as the team is very understaffed. You have missed teaching twice before due to this, and if you miss many more you are at risk of jeopardising progression to FY2.

Choose the **THREE most appropriate** *actions to take in this situation*

a) Explain that your session is compulsory and you really need to go

b) Accept the fact the you are in a difficult situation and not much can be done at the moment

c) Do as many tasks as you can before teaching and then leave for an hour

d) Inform the Foundation Programme Director of this problem

e) Call the education department and seek their advice

f) Stay on the ward as demanded by your registrar. However, attend the last half an hour of the session so at least you don't miss the whole session and you get the handout

g) As this is an ongoing problem, arrange for a friend to record future teaching sessions

h) Notify your consultant about the registrar's unfair demands

Practice Paper

3

Answers

Question 1: Wedding day

This scenario assesses the junior doctor's commitment to professionalism, ability to cope with pressure, communicate effectively, prioritise patient care appropriately and his / her skills in planning and organisation.

This scenario is unfortunately based on the experiences of a number of trainees. It is important to inform the staffing department as soon as you know you need time off and update them as soon as anything changes. Situations change and many things are beyond your control. Hopefully, the staffing department will match your conscientiousness and they will try and accommodate your needs as much as safe staffing levels allow. The New Doctor states:

'F1 doctors must demonstrate knowledge of their responsibilities to look after their health, including maintaining a suitable balance between work and personal life, and knowing how to deal with personal illness to protect patients.' (The New Doctor, paragraph 12).

A trainee can reasonably expect to be given annual leave for their wedding, especially when good notice is given.

The correct ranking of options in this scenario is:

D.A.C.B.E.

D - Inform your consultant

In this situation the first thing to do is inform the consultant responsible for your team of the situation and what you plan to do about it as they will need to know about any potential shortfalls in manpower. Also, once the situation is explained, your consultant should support you in your correspondence with the staffing department and your efforts to arrange suitable cover.

A - Remind medical staffing of your previous email correspondence and inform them that you will be taking the leave and ask them to help you find a swap

This option is the next most appropriate choice as it reflects confidence and an ability to work together in a difficult situation. A respectful, but firm, conversation with the staffing department should be undertaken to see if the issue can be resolved. The trainee must treat all colleagues fairly and with respect (Good Medical Practice, paragraph 36) and as such has the right to expect to be treated the same way. It is superior to options B and C, both of which result in you accepting the unfair situation without any attempt to highlight the main issue at hand.

C - Accept the rota and try to arrange swaps at a weeks' notice

In such circumstances one needs to attempt to address the main issue (the staffing department's poor handling of your leave issue) and this option does not attempt to do this. As there is an attempt to urgently find another person to swap your duties with, this has been ranked above option B.

B - Accept the rota and rearrange your wedding at a week's notice

This option is probably unworkable in practice and if it were necessary, would almost certainly undermine the trainee's relationship with the hospital in general, even if it does ensure that the team is appropriately staffed.

E - Make a formal complaint about medical staffing

It is very likely that pursuing the complaints avenue will take time and will not address the issue. Making a complaint may prevent similar episodes from taking place in the future, but the priority in this case is to take actions to ensure the leave is secured, and thus, this option has been ranked last.

Question 2: Reversing the Liverpool Care Pathway?

The Liverpool Care Pathway (LCP) is an integrated pathway designed to deliver holistic care to the dying patient. Its main aim is to keep the patient as comfortable and symptom free as possible. Patients are commenced on the LCP when it is thought that their prognosis is very poor and where active treatment will have little or no further benefit. All active ('curative') treatment is usually stopped when the decision is taken to commence the LCP. This decision is usually made in partnership with the patient (if possible) and their family. Most people on the LCP pass away within days, however, there are a minority of patients who recover from their 'terminal illness' and others who remain alive for longer than originally anticipated.

The correct ranking of options in this scenario is:

B.E.D.A.C.

B - Seek advice from the registrar from the other respiratory team (who is not involved in the patient's day-to-day care)

This is the best option as placing a patient on the LCP is a very sensitive decision that is made by a senior clinician, thus, re-examining the accuracy of the original decision in the new circumstance and considering a 'possible reversal' of that decision needs to be made by a senior doctor. The fact that the registrar does not know the patient's history is of secondary importance, as he will be able to acquaint himself with the patient's medical history from the patient's notes as well as from your input.

E - Perform a thorough review of the patient and make a decision based on that

This is a flawed option as it does not involve a senior clinician (one needs to recognise their own limitations particularly in complex and sensitive cases such as this one – Good Medical Practice, paragraph 14). It still attempts to address the pressing need of the situation, albeit in a deficient way, as a decision is being made based on the patient's current state. Thus, it is superior to option A where no attempt is made to reassess the patient; and option D, which critically overlooks the immediate nature of the concerns raised by the patient's daughter, and defers the situation on for a further two days, which is an unacceptable length of time to endure in this scenario.

D - Tell the daughter that the consultant who made the decision will be around in two days time and he is the most appropriate person to make a decision

All the remaining options are very poor. Option D has been selected above options A and C because options A and C both make very major decisions without any attempt to assess the patient. This option is nonetheless poor, as a two-day delay for the issue to be addressed in such a circumstance in unacceptable.

A - Restart antibiotic treatment as the patient is still alive after nine days

As above.

C - Tell the daughter that as the patient has been on the LCP for so many days, it is not in his best interest to stop it

This is the least favourable option as you have commented that recommencing active treatment is against the patient's best interest without even reviewing the patient to assess whether there has been significant change/improvement in his condition. There are numerous cases where patients who have been placed on the LCP improve sufficiently for active treatment to be recommended.

Question 3: You made the nurse cry

This scenario examines the junior doctor's ability to prioritise effectively, especially when dealing with unwell patients (who are the number one priority). It also assesses the doctor's ability to deal with the other members of the MDT effectively.

The correct ranking of options in this scenario is:

C.B.D.E.A.

C - Explain to the nurse again that the reason you could not complete the chart is because you are busy

This option demonstrates common courtesy and addresses the most immediate need that faces you in an effective and timely manner. As you have caused her sufficient distress to make her cry, it is very important to re-explain why you could not write the drug chart. You must apologise for hurting her feelings too. This will take less than a minute and given the fact that the nurse is in front of you and you have caused her to cry, it has been placed above option B. Furthermore, you will require the assistance of the nursing staff to assess and manage your unwell patient, the effectiveness of your teamwork will be significantly restricted if you have just left one of the nurses crying without apologising to her.

The GMC state in the Good Medical Practice (paragraph 59):

'You must not unfairly discriminate against patients or colleagues by allowing your personal views to affect your professional relationships or the treatment you provide or arrange. You should challenge colleagues if their behaviour does not comply with this guidance...'

B - Proceed to review your patient

Attending to the unwell patient will be the primary focus before attending to less urgent tasks, thus this is the most favourable option after C.

D - Hand the task over to the night team

Here you are taking responsibility for a task that is the responsibility of the medical team, and while not completing it yourself, you are making arrangements to get the task completed.

E - Ask the nurse to call the night team to re-write the chart

Option D is the better option as you have taken responsibility for the task, which is not a nursing duty, however, with this option you are still directing her towards a solution.

A - Re-write the drug chart

This option is poor as rewriting the chart is not a priority because you have two unwell patients who are waiting to be seen.

Question 4: Wrong dose and the patient has gone home

This scenario assesses the junior doctor's focus of patient care, utilisation of the MDT and recognising their own limitations.

The correct ranking of options in this scenario is:

A.D.C.B.E.

A - Ask the pharmacist about the adverse effects of the medication

The most important priority is to find out if the incorrect dose of this medication is dangerous or if it has the potential for significant side effects. Thus, utilising the pharmacist's skills to ascertain this information is the best first step; this is especially the case in this scenario as the pharmacist is next to you. The GMC state:

'You must be open and honest with patients if things go wrong. If a patient under your care has suffered harm or distress, you should:

a put matters right (if that is possible)

b offer an apology

c explain fully and promptly what has happened and the likely short-term and long-term effects'. (Good Medical Practice, paragraph 55).

D - Call your consultant to seek advice

Ideally you should not need to call your consultant about this, and it would be better to discuss the matter with the pharmacist. However, option D is superior to option C, as you are making a more informed decision.

C - Phone the patient and ask him to miss the next three doses and inform him of the correct dose

This is a sensible suggestion, however, it is wiser to make a more informed judgement, so options A and D are superior. Clinical judgement would lead you to make the decision that at present, re-admission to hospital is not indicated in the given context - as in option B.

B - Call the patient and ask him to come back

Based on the scenario, there is no indication to bring the patient back into hospital at this point and doing so will be an overreaction.

E - Tell the pharmacist not to worry as you reviewed the patient a few hours ago and he was absolutely fine

This option has the potential to harm the patient, and disregards the mistake, thus is the least favourable option.

Question 5: Racial abuse on the ward

This scenario deals with exercising good judgement in escalating matters, effective teamwork as well as the importance of patient consent.

The correct answers to this question are:

B.C.A.D.E.

B - Tell them that there's nothing much you can do and advice them to call security right away

This is the most appropriate option as it realises your personal limitations to help resolve the situation and directs the nurses towards appropriate escalation. While it would have been commendable to be more active in ones support of colleagues (as is the case in option C), the fact that you suggest security be called increases the likelihood of the problem being resolved, and thus makes this option superior to option C.

C - Confront the patient and tell him that this type of behavior is unacceptable

In this option you may not be contributing much to the situation in terms of overall outcome, however, there may be a possibility that the patient is more responsive to a doctor, over a nurse. Option B is superior as appropriate and effective escalation is being suggested. This option also supports good teamwork, thus is ranked second.

A - Do nothing, as you are quite busy and it is not your problem, there are also plenty of nurses there already

While your response to the nurses may not be incorrect, it has an element of 'indifference' that is not conducive to good teamwork. The fact that it is the nurse being abused does not mean 'it is not your problem'. The GMC strongly emphasises the importance of working well within a team and supporting colleagues who have problems. However, this option is superior to D and E as explained below.

D - Tell the patient to leave the hospital as NHS staff are not to be treated in this manner

It is true that NHS staff cannot be treated in this manner, but to tell the patient to leave before assessing the situation holistically, for example, by excluding the possibility that the patient may be confused, is premature and does not promote good care.

E - Prescribe some haloperidol to calm the patient down

Prescribing sedatives without the patient's expressed consent, and simply because he is 'rowdy', is not acceptable and may be seen as assaulting the patient.

Consent is necessary whenever a patient who has mental capacity is examined, investigated or treated. All patients are deemed to have capacity unless it has been demonstrated otherwise (as determined by the Mental Capacity Act 2005). There are three main elements to valid consent; a) – it needs to be given by a patient who has capacity, b) – the consent needs to be voluntary without any undue influence, and c) – sufficient amount of information should be provided about the procedure (informed consent). It is not lawful to administer medical treatment (to a competent patient) without consent and it may be seen as a criminal offence. (See the GMC's guidance on consent for further details).

Question 6: Family kept waiting

This scenario assesses the junior doctor's judgements on work-life balance, prioritisation and communication. The GMC's guidance state that *'you must be considerate to those close to the patient and be sensitive and responsive in giving them information and support....'. (Good Medical Practice, paragraph 33).* In doing this you must follow the GMC's guidance on 'Confidentiality: Protecting and providing information'.

The correct ranking of options in this scenario is:

C.E.D.B.A.

C - Explain to the family that you have been very busy with unwell patients and you can't talk to them today

This is the best option as you are being honest with the family and you are explaining the reason why you cannot have the discussion today. It is also fair on yourself, as this is a task that can wait and is not urgent, and you should not be doing non-urgent tasks so late after your shift has ended – see The New Doctor paragraph 12 on work-life balance.

E - Give the family a quick five minute summary and tell them you will address any concerns they have tomorrow

This is a good option, however, it has not been ranked first as a 'five-minute' conversation can easily turn into a '20 minute' discussion in this context (where the family have been waiting for a long time), thus it has been ranked second. A discussion about the patient's 'complex needs' should not be rushed, and the family should be given time to express their thoughts and concerns. Therefore, stating that you will discuss their concerns tomorrow is wise.

D - Inform the family that you will speak to them tomorrow

This option acts to resolve the issue by arranging another appropriate time to sit and discuss the matter with the family. However, you have not explained to the family why you could not talk to them on that very same day, unlike in option C. Option E also does not provide a reason for the delay in holding the discussion with the family, but it does leave them with a basic update in addition to a further discussion on the next day, thus it has been ranked above option D.

B - Sit down with the family and have a discussion with them

This is not a good prioritisation of tasks as the discussion with the family can wait and is not urgent. Furthermore, you have a responsibility for your own wellbeing, so to perform non-urgent tasks three hours after your shift has ended is not desirable.

A - Avoid the family on your way out as it is already very late and they may start talking to you

This is unprofessional behaviour, and it is unfair on the relatives as they have been waiting a long time to talk to you.

Question 7: Attending your prize award ceremony

This scenario assesses the junior doctor's ability to prioritise effectively, focus on patient care, deal with difficult situations and understand the basic working procedures in a surgical team.
The correct ranking of options in this scenario is:

B.C.A.D.E.

B & C - (B) Go to the A&E department and explain your situation to the registrar & (C) Call your registrar again and tell him that you need to leave

Both these options do the most appropriate thing by informing the registrar of the situation. This is very important for many reasons, especially as he is planning to come up to the ward in a little while to review the patient. Option B supersedes option C as you are explaining the situation rather than 'telling him that you need to leave'. Furthermore, going to A&E and explaining in person is preferred, this will be more effective as the registrar is on-call and his bleep is ringing constantly and it has already been difficult to contact him via his bleep. Also, the scenario informed you that you have had difficulties in reaching him already. It is important to state that your desire to leave will not compromise patient care, as you have correctly prioritised the unwell patient, performed all the investigations and commenced management prior to wanting to leave.

A - Call the on-call house officer and handover the patient to him/her

This is the normal course of action to follow when an important task needs to be completed in the evening.

'F1 doctors must work effectively as a member of a team, including supporting others, handover and taking over the care

of a patient safely and effectively from other health professionals.' (The New Doctor, paragraph 10).

This option, however, disregards the registrar who is expecting to come up and review the patient with you, and thus is ranked third.

D - Try to find a different registrar to review the patient

This is an unwise decision for many reasons, most importantly because you have already discussed the patient with your registrar who has already advised on a management plan. It is not sensible to try and involve another registrar who will not be familiar with this patient. Furthermore, it is after normal working times, so finding another registrar to review the patient will not be very easy.

E - Put the patient on the 'night handover' so he is seen by a doctor later, and leave

This is the least favourable option as it contravenes patient care by leaving the unwell patient without senior review for many hours. It also disregards the registrar.

Question 8: Skiving off the post take round

This scenario deals with probity, professionalism and patient care.

The correct ranking of options in this scenario is:

C.B.E.D.A.

C - Express your feelings to her and come up with an appropriate solution

This is the most favourable response, as you will help prevent a similar situation from happening again by expressing your feelings to the colleague. It also leads to an 'appropriate' resolution of the problem.

B - Inform her registrar of what has happened

This is an acceptable and suitable level of escalation given what has happened. In circumstances where a colleague's behaviour is likely to negatively impact patients' care, the GMC advice that you raise your concerns in an honest manner: *'If you have concerns that a colleague may not be fit to practise and may be putting patients at risk, you must ask for advice from a colleague, your defence body or us. If you are still concerned you must report this, in line with our guidance and your workplace policy, and make a record of the steps you have taken.' (Good Medical Practice, paragraph 25c).*

E - Inform your consultant of the situation and suggest that your colleague should be asked to help your team during your next post take ward round

Is a less favourable option as you are prioritising the fact that you have been treated unfairly by your colleague's absence over the fact that what she did impacted patient care in a negative way and was unprofessional and dishonest. It has been ranked above options D and A as you are still escalating the situation to a senior, albeit the inappropriate clinician, as your consultant is not responsible for the colleague in question.

D - As this has only happened once, do nothing

This is a poor option, as it contravenes patient care. This is because the colleague's unprofessional and dishonest behaviour has left the team short staffed and this will naturally have an impact on the level of care that can be provided to patients. The GMC state:

'You must support colleagues who have problems with their performance or health. But you must put patient safety first at all times.' (Good Medical Practice, paragraph 43).

A - Ask the colleague to cover some of your on-calls to make up

This is the least favourable option as there is no real attempt to address the problem and prevent the situation from re-arising. One can argue that her behaviour is being implicitly condoned and your request that she cover your on-calls constitutes blackmail.

Question 9: Can't get work off my mind

This scenario assesses the prioritisation of patient care in an appropriate manner and understanding of basic procedures and processes in a medical team.

The correct ranking of options in this scenario is:

C.B.D.A.E.

C - Phone the ward nurses from home and ask them to check that the catheter is okay

This is the most favourable option as it addresses the situation in a prompt and appropriate manner. The nurse taking care of the patient is in an ideal position to check that there are no problems.

B - Phone the night SHO covering the wards and ask her to check that the catheter is okay

This is the second best option as similarly to option C, the patient is assessed promptly. However, the night SHO will most probably be busy with many other duties and thus will take longer to respond, hence option C has been preferred.

D - Go back to hospital to check on the patient, as you were the one who placed the catheter in

While this ensures the patient is attended to promptly, and thus placed above options A and E, it is unnecessary for you to go back to hospital to perform this task which can be carried out by another member of staff. Options C, B and D all address the problem at hand promptly, keeping with the key GMC principle to make the care of your patient your first concern (Good Medical Practice, paragraph 1).

A - Check that the patient is well and there are no complications with the catheter first thing next morning

In this option there is a significant delay in attending to the patient and thus there is an increased risk of paraphimosis developing if the foreskin is left retracted. This option contravenes patient care and has been ranked low.

E - Call the patient's team the next day to ensure that the patient is well and does not have any problems

This is the least favourable option as you have waited till the next day, furthermore your enquiry to the team is very vague. It is also better for you ensure that the patient has no complications since you are in hospital and it was you who catheterised the patient.

Question 10: Too many referrals!

This scenario assesses the junior doctor's ability to deal with pressure and their problem solving attributes.

The correct ranking of options in this scenario is:

C.D.B.E.A.

C - Call the consultant surgeon at his home phone, through the switchboard, and ask him to resolve the problem

This is the most important thing to do as there is a critical problem, and it is the consultant on-call who is ultimately responsible for the acute surgical admissions for that day. It is his responsibility to address this situation with the urgency required. The GMC state that in providing a good standard of practice and care, you must *'Recognise and work within the limits of your competence; Work with colleagues in the ways that best serve patients' interests.'* *(Good Medical Practice, duties of a doctor).*

D - Discuss the situation with the A&E registrar and ask him to deal with the surgical patients for the time being

This is similar to B, however, superior as most of your patients will be referred by A&E, thus explaining the situation to the A&E SpR will yield two immediate benefits - you will not get A&E referrals till this issue is resolved, and also, he may advise you on how best to resolve the situation.

B - Reject all incoming referrals explaining the situation to the caller

This approach is safer than the options below as at this point, the patients who get accepted by the surgical team will not have a surgeon to review them. Furthermore, your team is severely understaffed, and you will most probably not be able to attend to the needs of the patients being referred on to you. Thus, it is best for the current team to continue their care until the seniors in the surgical team become available again.

E - Accept the referrals explaining that you are the only team member around for the time being

This is an unfavourable option as you are accepting patients who you, and your absent team, will not be able to attend to for an unspecified amount of time - this contravenes patient care. It is better for the patient to receive 'some medical care' under their current team than to be accepted by the surgical team who will be unable to meet their care need at the present time.

A - Turn your bleep off for half an hour as it is stressing you out

This is a very poor option, as it does not help address the situation, now the entire surgical team is unavailable! This will lead to a greater degree of confusion and adversely affect patient safety by delaying a resolution to the problem.

Question 11: Just trying to relax with your flatmates

This scenario assesses the junior doctor's understanding of confidentiality, as well as their dealing with patients' relatives.

The correct ranking of options in this scenario is:

B.D.E.A.C.

B - Explain to the relative that the earliest you can discuss the patient's care is tomorrow morning

This is the best course to take as you do not disclose information to the relative without the patient's permission; furthermore, you address the situation by offering another time to discuss the patient's health.

'Confidentiality is central to trust between doctors and patients. Without assurances about confidentiality, patients may be reluctant to seek medical attention or to give doctors the information they need in order to provide good care.' (GMC confidentiality guidance, paragraph 6).

D - Advise the relative that the nurse taking care of the patient would be the best point of call at this time

This is a favourable option as it passes responsibility to a member of staff on the ward who is 'on duty'. As the patient's medical team is unavailable at present, the next best avenue for updates is the nursing staff. Option B has been selected over this as the team doctor is in a better position to discuss the questions that are being raised.

E - Ask the relative to hand the phone over to the colleague who gave them your number and reprimand her for giving out your number without asking you first

This does not address the needs of the situation and thus has been ranked low. It has been placed above option A as it is unfair for you to express your grievances to the patient's relative. The GMC state that *'you must be considerate to those close to the patient and be sensitive and responsive in giving them information and support....'. (Good Medical Practice, paragraph 33).*

A - Tell the relative it is your private line and you won't be speaking to him now, and that your colleague made a big mistake in giving him your number

This option has been ranked fourth as it is unfair to express your grievances to the relative like that. While your feelings of frustration are understandable, it is not the relative who is at fault, rather the colleague who gave out your private number.

C - Have a quick discussion with the relative and say that you can provide more details tomorrow

This is the least favourable option as you do not know for sure who you are speaking to, and more importantly you do not know if the patient is happy for you to disclose his medical details.

Question 12: Final year student lets slip

This scenario assesses the junior doctor's communication skills, honesty in dealing with patients and the ability to handle difficult situations.

The correct ranking of options in this scenario is:

D.E.A.C.B.

D - Tell the patient that the medical team will answer her questions after the CT scan is done

This is the most honest and appropriate answer, even if it does not leave the patient fully at ease. This is ranked first as it is the same response that the senior members of your team would give the patient, as they do not have any more information than you do. Of relevance is that all of the answers are less than ideal, as you need to listen to the patient's concerns and reassure her in an honest manner as well as inform her that you will be able to disclose more information after the CT scan. The question assesses your ability to distinguish between the options provided.

E - Inform the patient that the consultant is doing a ward round tomorrow and she will be able to answer any questions that the patient has

This helps alleviate some anxieties as you have said that the consultant will address her concerns tomorrow. However, option D is preferable, as you have given a more specific update without waiting for the consultant, who will also have to wait for the CT scan results. Furthermore, there is a one-day delay in the consultant speaking to the patient.

A - Advise the medical student that he should not have made the remark

This action is appropriate and needs to be done to prevent the student from making the same mistake again, but it does not serve to address the key needs of the situation and thus is ranked low. The Good Medical Practice states:

'You should be prepared to contribute to teaching and training doctors and students.' (Paragraph 39).

This option has, however, been ranked above options C and B as has been explained below.

C - Phone your registrar and ask her to come up from clinic to update the patient on the current situation

This is not a wise option as there is not much more that the registrar can explain to the patient at this point. You are also 'calling her up to the ward' from her other duties in a situation where her input would be restricted, as the CT scan has not happened yet. Furthermore, in hospital settings you will constantly be faced with challenging situations, you need to demonstrate initiative in dealing with them.

B - Reassure the patient telling her that she'll be fine

This is the least favourable option as the patient is being given dishonest reassurance. Patients have the right to know about their health, and thus providing false reassurance is incorrect.

Question 13: Colleague gone AWOL

This scenario assesses the junior doctor's commitment to patient care, prioritisation of patient safety and understanding of the European Working Time Directive (EWTD). The EWTD gives European workers specific rights in relation to their working hours and shifts. Amongst other rules, it demands a rest period of at least 11 continuous hours in any 24 hour period.

The correct ranking of options in this scenario is:

C.A.B.D.E.

C - Tell the registrar that you'll hold the bleep for a further half an hour

This is the best option as you are assisting the registrar in dealing with this problem, and, at the same time, you have given him a specific and reasonable amount of time in which to address the matter. This is important as you have just completed a long shift and you are not functioning at your optimum level, and thus are more prone to mistakes. Furthermore, it is not fair on you to work long after you have just completed your 12-hour shift.

A - Hold the bleep and wait for the registrar to address the issue, or for the locum to arrive

Here you are helping the situation; but it is less favourable than C where you specify to the registrar how long you will stay and by doing so, emphasise the need for the problem to be addressed as soon as possible.

B - Explain to the registrar that you have just completed a long shift and can't hold onto the bleep

In this option you have decided not to help in this difficult situation where a small amount of your time will help the team quite significantly, thus this is less favourable than C and A. However, it is preferable to option D as you are giving a clear reason why you are unable to help.

D - Suggest that the register would be able to cope with the SHO bleep for a little while as the last few hours have been very quiet

This option is similar to B and does not help the situation. In addition to that, your response to the SpR is quite unconstructive.

E - Offer to cover the night shift on the condition that you are paid locum rates for your services

This is the least desirable option as it is bad for patient care. Firstly, because it is the SHO bleep, and you are an FY1 and thus you should not take on a responsibility beyond your competency. Secondly, because you will function at a sub-optimal level after completing your 12-hour long shift. The GMC state that *'you must recognise and work within the limits of your competence.' (Good Medical Practice, paragraph 14).*

Question 14: Patient fed up and wants to go home

This scenario assesses the junior doctor's ability to prioritise tasks and make decisions based on patients' needs and their care.

The correct ranking of options in this scenario is:

B.E.A.D.C.

B - Explain to the patient that her latest investigations have shown abnormal results and the consultant will confirm these findings with her

This is the best first step as it gives the patient a clear reason why she needs to stay for a little while longer without disclosing all the news (the benefits of not disclosing all the news have been explained below). Furthermore, you inform the patient that she can expect further details from the consultant. This option has been ranked above Option E as it addresses the needs of the situation in a more immediate manner, as it is likely that the consultant or registrar will be unable to come straightaway and break the news, even after the situation is explained to them.

E - Find out if your consultant or registrar can break the news any sooner

This is a good option given the fact that the patient wishes to leave hospital. If option B does not suffice, this is the next best way to help her make an informed decision.

A - Break the news to the patient and tell her that she needs to stay for some further tests

It is not ideal for FY1 doctors to be breaking news of cancer diagnoses, especially as they will be less well equipped to discuss 'what happens next', including the details of the different options that are available to the patient. This, however, is still a good option as it will help persuade the patient to reconsider her decision by making an informed decision based on new facts.

D - Call a family member and ask them to persuade the patient to stay, explaining to them the latest diagnosis

This is very unfavourable as it breaches the patient's confidentiality despite the apparent benefit of persuading her to stay in hospital. It has been ranked above option C, as it will not have as negative an effect on her health as option C.

C - Offer her a 'discharge against medical advice form'

This is a very poor option as no attempt is made to provide the patient with an understanding of why it is important to remain in hospital. Thus, offering her the discharge against medical advice form without explaining the current state of affairs contributes very negatively to her care.

Question 15: FY2 intruding

This scenario deals with patient care, communication skills, confidentiality and teamwork. It is important to realise that the FY2 in this scenario is not involved in the patient's care and is not present at the ward rounds/MDT meetings; and thus may lack a clear picture about the patient's care. Furthermore, the FY2's behaviour may undermine the medical team caring for the patient.

The correct ranking of options in this scenario is:

A.B.C.E.D.

A - Speak to the FY2 in question and request he stops communicating each entry in the notes to the relatives

This is the most sensible option as if it is done politely, it should not hurt the feelings of the doctor, nor will it place the family in an awkward position by asking them not to take updates from their friend. It is the option that has the best potential to resolve the situation easily.

B - Discuss the problem with your registrar and ask him to speak to the FY2

This is also a good option, as your SpR is senior to the doctor in question he will be better placed to discuss the issue with the doctor if he feels it appropriate.

C - Explain politely to the patient's relatives that the medical team are the best point of call for any enquiries they may have

A and B are preferred over this option as it is not the family who are at fault here, furthermore, the family may get slightly offended by the indirect request not to receive updates from the other doctor, their friend.

E - Contact the FY2's registrar and request that she ask him to stop coming up the ward
This is very harsh as one should not need to resort to this to solve the problem. The demand that he does not come up to the ward is also excessive.

D - Let the FY2 continue as he is, as it is not harming the patient in any way

This is the least favourable question as it impinges on patient's confidentiality. The FY2 from the other team is not providing medical care to the patient and thus should not be looking at confidential details about the patient's care. Furthermore, the patient's consent is required for this information to be imparted to the family. The FY2's frequent visits also impinge on your ability to work well as you are being regularly questioned about the patient's progress.

Question 16: Reprimanded for minor error

This scenario assesses the junior doctor's ability to prioritise patient care and work effectively in a team. The Good Medical Practice gives clear guidance on how to act when a patient has suffered distress (paragraph 55). You must also *'support colleagues who have problems with their performance or health. But you must put patient safety first at all times' (paragraph 43)* and *'you must not unfairly discriminate against patients or colleagues by allowing your personal views to affect your professional relationships or the treatment you provide or arrange. You should challenge colleagues if their behaviour does not comply with this guidance...' (paragraph 59).*

The correct ranking of options in this scenario is:

A.E.B.C.D.

A & E - (A) Rectify the minor error & (E) Reassure the patient and tell her not to worry

As patient care is priority number one, it is most important to 'undo the error' and reassure the patient.

B - Reassure the FY2 and tell him that it was actually quite a minor thing and the registrar over reacted

This is important after attending to the needs of the patient, especially as it involves a fellow junior member of the team and your reassurance will help their confidence.

C - Talk to your registrar explaining that it would have been better to give the criticism in private

It is important to tell your registrar that it would have been best to correct the FY2 when the other members of the MDT and the patient were not present, as there is a chance that the SpR may have overlooked that. However, as the SpR is senior to both of you, it could be difficult in certain cases to give this important feedback.

D - Inform your consultant of what has happened

As the scenario makes no mention that this is a recurrent problem, there is no indication to get the consultant involved. The team should be able to resolve this without resorting to escalating to the consultant (at this stage).

Question 17: A kind gesture

This scenario raises the complexities attached to accepting gifts from patients.

The GMC state:

'You must not ask for or accept – from patients, colleagues or others – any inducement, gift or hospitality that may affect or be

seen to affect the way you prescribe for, treat or refer patients or commission services for patients. You must not offer these inducements.' (Good Medical Practice, paragraph 80).

The correct ranking of options in this scenario is:

C.E.D.A.B.

C - Tell him it would be better to add it to the ward fund instead

It is common practice that when a patient offers a gift within a hospital setting, the gift is encouraged to go towards the ward. This is in keeping with the GMC guidelines stated above. This action implies that you were not the only one involved in the patient's care. It also sets a precedence for any similar future occurrence.

E - Tell him a thank-you card would do

Sometimes the patient will be especially grateful for your specific care, and insist on giving you a gift. For this reason, option E is the most appropriate way of discouraging the gift whilst maintaining an appreciation for the patient's gesture.

D - Tell him that £50 is too much and if anything to give you half of that

Options D and A are extremely similar, however, option D is preferred over option A because it demonstrates a greater gesture of discouragement (in accepting the gift) than option A, where it is readily accepted.

A - Thank him for his generosity and accept his gift

The complexities of accepting gifts, especially monetary gifts, from patients have been communicated by the GMC guidelines stated above. The guidelines are clear in that accepting gifts should not be encouraged, however, nowhere does it state that it is prohibited.

B - Refuse the money and state it is against rules

To this end, refusal of gifts based on it being 'against the rules' is untrue and may even be seen as an abrupt and unkind response to a patient's token of gratitude, specifically in this case where the patient is insistent.

Question 18: All I'm asking for is to go to theatres

This scenario deals with teamwork, communication skills, teaching and learning and appropriate levels of escalation.

The correct ranking of options in this scenario is:

C.D.A.B.E.

C - Sit down with the SHO and explain how you feel

This is the most appropriate thing to do in this situation. There are no signs of mal-intent from the SHO, and by you politely expressing your feelings to the SHO it is very likely an amicable solution can be agreed upon. This is the best first step.

D - Ask the registrar to discuss the situation with the SHO

This is the second best option and it is preferred to options B and A as it will address the situation in a 'non-confrontational manner'. It is preferable to escalate to the team registrar in this situation as it would still be a 'more informal channel' to deal with the issue as the registrar is not responsible for the SHO's final assessments.

A & B – (A) Voice your concerns to your consultant that there is an unfair distribution of the ward duties & (B) Ask your educational supervisor to talk to the SHO

Both these options are similar and less than ideal, as an attempt should be made to address the situation using simpler methods first. Furthermore, escalating to the consultants in the first instant can cause a rift between you and the SHO. Option A is preferred over option B, as your consultant would be the more appropriate person to raise this issue with.

E - Go to theatres for a few hours, directly after the ward round and then return to do your jobs

This is not a good method to apply and will affect patient care in a negative way as essential tasks will get delayed, thus this is the least favourable option.

Question 19: Parents will 'have a go'

This scenario deals with issues of confidentiality and consent. For patients who are under 16, you have to consider if the child has Fraser Competence to determine whether the child is able to consent to medical treatment without the need for parental permission or knowledge. The child in this case is 16 years old and has full rights to confidentiality.

The correct ranking of options in this scenario is:

B.A.E.D.C.

B - Respect the patient's wishes, but explain that you feel it is in his best interest to inform his parents

This is the best option as it preserves confidentiality. As the patient is 16 years old his confidentiality must be respected. This option also makes an attempt to assess the situation and address it by encouraging the patient to discuss the issues with his parents.

A - Accept his wishes and tell him you won't mention it to his parents

This respects his wishes and complies with the rules; however, there are potential negative implications to his health if you simply leave the matter here without exploring it further (as it is hiding the problem, rather than addressing it). Encouraging him to discuss the issue with those around him *may* be better for him in the long-term).

E - Call the diabetic nurse to come and speak to the patient

This is a good option as the diabetic nurse will have a greater level of expertise in this situation and can discuss other options that the patient can consider to help his problem such as patient support groups. It is less relevant to the immediate needs of the situation and thus has been ranked third. As it does not breach confidentiality, it is naturally preferable to options D and C.

D - Phone the head teacher of the school and explain the situation

Informing the school is important as the problem relates to the patient being at school. However, this option breaks confidentiality as there is no mention of seeking the patient's permission. It is also less relevant to the acute needs of the situation. It has been preferred over option C as the patient has clearly and specifically stated that his parents are not to be informed, so the breach in confidentiality is more emphatic in option C.

C - Inform his parents as they have parental responsibility over him

This breaches confidentiality, especially against the patient's expressed wishes for his patents not to be told, and thus is not the correct thing to do. As the patient is now 16 years old, he is able to make his own decisions and his parents do not have that 'responsibility' any longer.

Question 20: Squeamish patient & the blood cultures

This question assesses multiple characteristics required of a foundation year doctor. The scenario ties together the need to recognise mistakes and seek help when necessary, communicate effectively and be honest and open with patients. The GMC Good Medical Practice guidelines state as the primary duty of a doctor:

'Make the care of your patient your first concern'

To this end, the optimal order for the scenario would be:

B.A.E.D.C.

B - Return and apologise to the patient for your mistake and offer to take blood again

The most important aspect being tested is the requirement of a junior doctor to act with honesty and integrity. While it would be perfectly reasonable to ask a colleague to perform the procedure instead, it is vital to maintain the doctor-patient trust. The following paragraph from the Good Medical Practice outlines the appropriate initial response within such a scenario.

'You must be open and honest with patients if things go wrong. If a patient under your care has suffered harm or distress, you should:

a put matters right (if that is possible)

b offer an apology

c explain fully and promptly what has happened and the likely short-term and long-term effects.'

(Good Medical Practice, paragraph 55).

A - Ask a nurse to return and take bloods again

It is quite understandable if the doctor is embarrassed or hesitant to have a few more attempts to get the blood culture, especially in a patient who is very reluctant to be bled anyway. One may not be incorrect to assume that the patient may have more confidence in a different member of staff, and thus, seeking help from a colleague may be beneficial both for the patient and the doctor, who would naturally feel more pressurised by the situation. While this option is very reasonable, the fact that there is no mention of apologising to the patient and informing him of what has happened means that it is not the best option to follow.

E - Inform the laboratory of the situation and ask them to consider the non-sterile conditions when analysing the bottles you are due to send

Phoning the laboratory and getting their feedback on the situation would not be a bad call. It is very likely that the lab will request new samples, but this approach still demonstrates a reasonable effort by the junior doctor to assess the situation and work towards the correct solution.

D - Bleep your registrar and inform him of the situation

It is important for the junior doctor to consult with senior members of the team when needed, however, calling the registrar at this point is a poor decision to make. No attempt has yet been made by the junior doctor to establish the significance of the problem or rectify it. Junior doctors are expected to be capable of drawing blood safely and by sterile means. If one is unable to take blood for whatever reason, then one should work up the colleague ladder before asking the registrar. If other avenues have been exhausted, it may not be so unreasonable to seek the registrar's advice and support, but not at this stage.

C - Send the bloods off anyway as the laboratory should be able to distinguish between pneumonia-causing pathogens and anything else that may have been caught from the patient's bedside

Sending non-sterile bottles to the laboratory can have a negative effect on the patient's diagnosis and subsequent management, and must be avoided. This option would also have a negative effect on doctor-patient trust.

Question 21: Dealing with death

This question assesses how you respond to challenging situations. Being able to cope and work effectively under pressure is an essential quality required to function as a doctor. It assesses your ability to adapt to changing circumstances and manage uncertainties.

The most appropriate options are:

C.E.G.

C - Ask the senior nurse to take the family to a quiet room

E - Inform the family of the death

G - Ask the health care assistant to ensure the patient's body is in a dignified state

C&E - Option C and E are very important, as you are the only doctor available, you should assume responsibility and break the news to the family. It would be appropriate to gain help from the nurse and to usher the family into a quiet room, firstly to stop them coming onto the ward abruptly, and also to give you time to gather your thoughts before breaking the bad news. It is important to recognise that you are part of a team, both you and the nursing staff were delivering care to the patient. It is advisable therefore, to ask a nurse to be present, as she can provide support to not only the family, but to you as well. Creating an environment free of distractions, where full attention can be given to the family, is essential when breaking such sensitive news. In a circumstance where you were not able to break the bad news, the senior ward nurse would be a very appropriate person to break this news on behalf of the medical team.

G - This may not seem an obvious initial response, but will in fact have a big impact on the family. It will allow the family to see their loved one in a clean and dignified state. This is especially important as the patient has just passed away following a failed resuscitation attempt, and may have blood stains on his/her body, and may be connected to monitoring devices and intravenous lines.

'You must be considerate to those close to the patient and be sensitive and responsive in giving them information and support.' (Good Medical Practice, paragraph 33).

B - This is a fair response to the situation however is not of immediate concern, as the consultant wouldn't be able to impact the immediate situation from his clinic. Contacting him as a response to the scenario will yield limited benefit.

F - This does not address any of the immediate needs of the scenario and is not a priority. The true extent of the shortfall of doctors on the ward is also difficult to gauge given that the information provided in the scenario only concerns one particular day.

A - This is incorrect. While it would be more suitable for a more senior doctor to break such news, in this case you are the only doctor on the ward and hence need to take on this responsibility.

D - This is option is not ideal as it is unfair on the family to be left waiting while you try to find a senior doctor to break the bad news. As the scenario stated, all your seniors are unavailable at present and thus, the family may be left waiting for an unacceptable amount of time.

H - Although you must always be open about your role and limitations, this would be inappropriate as it could imply that the patient's demise was a result of a lack of senior doctors on the ward. It is important to note that the 'crash team' would have had senior doctors in it. There is no indication in the scenario that the patient's condition was affected by the absence of you senior team members.

Question 22: Lazy colleague

This question deals with many core competencies that are required of a doctor. You are being assessed on your ability to communicate effectively with colleagues, your problem solving skills and your ability to encourage a healthy working atmosphere.

The correct answers to this scenario are:

D.F.H.

D - Explore reasons for your colleague's attitude and offer support if required

F - Advise your colleague to attend work on time

H - Tell your colleague that his conduct is unfair and stressing you out

D - This is a correct option as it serves to explore or discuss the situation with your colleague as well as offer support if required. While it is important to advise your colleague (as is reflected in option F), you should also provide assistance and support where necessary, particularly as the colleague may have problems adversely impacting his ability to work effectively as a doctor. This is reflected in the Good Medical Practice guidance: *'You must support colleagues who have problems with their performance or health. But you must put patient safety first at all times.'* (Paragraph 43).

F - When faced with challenging working relationships, one must ensure that this does not compromise patient care. All effort should be made to address any tensions between team members in order to create an environment conducive to delivering optimal patient care. Any factors that are likely to affect patient care in a negative way must also be addressed in the appropriate manner. It may be that your colleague needs reminding about what is required of him, and a helpful reminder may be all that is needed.

H - This would serve to communicate to your colleague the consequences of his actions, emphasise the importance of addressing the issue, and will hopefully contribute to a positive change. The unequal distribution of work is an unjust burden on you, and you should work to correct it. While this option may serve to encourage your colleague to become more responsible, initial priority should still be to explore the reasons for his behaviour and provide support where necessary. This would serve to foster a healthy working environment.

A - This is a very harsh initial response, and one must attempt to address and resolve the issue with the colleague as a first step. If that were to prove unsuccessful, it would be reasonable to escalate to seniors.

B & G - Similarly to option A, these options can also be deemed as reasonable choices, however, it would be more advisable to initially approach your colleague directly, and if this doesn't prove successful, to then seek your registrar's assistance.

C - Similarly, this would be more appropriate only after you have taken steps to advise your colleague yourself. When raising any concerns, it is important to bear in mind that you do not unfairly discriminate against your colleague, as it would only serve to adversely affect the working relationship.

E - This would not be a healthy option as avoiding facing such issues would lead to a total breakdown in trust within the team. It will also contribute negatively to patient care.

Question 23: Heartbroken

The correct answers to this scenario are: **A.G.H.**

A - Inform the registrar on-call

G - Suggest she calls her seniors and lets them know of the situation

H - Discuss the staffing challenges with the other juniors on-call

A - Your primary concern should be to provide a good standard of practice and care for your patients and this may be negatively affected by having fewer doctors on-call. It is your responsibility to inform managers and seniors of the problem so they can organise cover for the rest of the day. At the same time, it is also your responsibility to support colleagues who have problems with performance, conduct or health.

G - It is the doctor's responsibility to work and communicate effectively with colleagues within and outside of the team. Therefore, it is primarily the responsibility of the doctor who is not able to fulfil the on-call commitment to inform medical staffing and his/her seniors. Hence option G will be the appropriate.

H - This option will ensure that you have tried your best to minimise the effects of one less staff by discussing the issue with other junior colleagues on-call. This will hopefully lead to reprioritisation and reorganisation of tasks to ensure that patient safety is not compromised.

C - This option is undesirable as it implies that you are not involving other colleagues, or making any plans to minimise the impact of the staff shortage (the importance of which has already been highlighted above).

D - Speaking to the clinical supervisor could be appropriate if you feel this is persistent problem. However, this course of action would not be necessary in the immediate setting.

B - Your colleague is a professional who has responsibility for her actions, thus it is her duty to discuss her difficulties with her seniors. It is not your role to be calling her and demanding that she come to work. The senior doctors will have to assess the issue and come to a decision on how best to address it.

E&F - Both these options demonstrate concern for your colleague, but the most pressing priority is to address the staff shortage in the busy on-call, thus these options have not been selected.

Question 24: 'It's a free country'

The correct answers to this scenario are: **A.B.G.**

A - Ask him to sign a document saying he understands the risks associated with leaving the ward

B - Emphasise the risks involved if he doesn't stay connected to the monitor

G - Respect the patient's decision. Let him come and go as he pleases

A & B & G - In this situation good communication is vital. It is of paramount importance to ensure the patient understands his condition and what risks he is exposing himself to by leaving the ward. You must also be confident that the patient has capacity to make the decisions he is making. There is no suggestion in this scenario that the patient has any issues that would limit his capacity to make decisions, thus it must be assumed that he has full capacity. If the patient decides not to adhere to medical advice and there are potentially adverse consequences to his actions, then it is good practice to get the patient to sign a form to state that he is refusing medical advice. It is important to point out that hospital is not a prison, and patients are free to leave should they wish, thus options C and D would be inappropriate.

E - As a principled first step, we must respect the patient's autonomy (G). As has been emphasised, medical professionals cannot enforce their recommendations on competent adults without consent. Asking the patients' relatives to persuade the patient to change his course of action may be an appropriate apporach, however, discussing 'the whole situation' with them would be a breach of confidentiality and must be avoided. It is also more worthy to approach the patient directly first (B), even if nurses have approached him before. Your duty is to outline the risks to the patient even if he has heard them elsewhere previously. As we are compelled to allow him to leave the ward due to the principle of autonomy, it would be very important that he signs a declaration saying he understands the risks of his actions (A). These actions may be followed on by option E. However, as has been explained, you will need to get the patient's agreement to discuss the situation with his family.

D - This is not appropriate as nurses are not assigned to care for one patient each (except in ITU), and by spending a vast amount of time with one uncooperative patient, they would be compromising care for many other patients.

H - This is a harsh approach to take and one should not be threatening patients in such a manner. This goes against Good Medical Practice guidelines:

'You must support patients in caring for themselves to empower them to improve and maintain their health. This may, for example, include:

a advising patients on the effects of their life choices and lifestyle on their health and well-being

b supporting patients to make lifestyle changes where appropriate...' (Paragraph 51).

Question 25: You lose your cool at the nurse

This scenario assesses the junior doctor's ability to deal with pressure, prioritise actions and function well as a part of a team. The GMC emphasise the importance of good teamwork and respect for colleagues in many different places in the Good Medical Practice guidelines.

The correct answer to this scenario: **A.B.H.**

A - Apologise to the nurse for putting the phone down on her

B - Hold your ground about not reviewing the rash yesterday as you had other priorities

H - Go and perform a detailed review of the patient and document your findings

A - It is important to apologise to the nurse for putting the phone down on her. Despite your grievances, which are very understandable, putting the phone down on her was a mistake and you should apologise in the spirit of good teamwork and in recognition of your error.

B - This option is very important, as often in hospitals you will have conflicting demands from various people. The scenario demonstrates that you prioritised your tasks with good judgement, and thus it is important that you stand by your judgement. This should be the case unless you are shown to have made an incorrect judgement.

H - This is a very important next step, as it prioritises the patient's needs over the disagreements within the MDT. The patient must be your first concern (Good Medical Practice). It also strengthens your standing should a complaint be made against you.

C - This option may be a viable option later on if this nurse persists in threatening to call your seniors whenever she wants something from you, but this is not implied in the scenario. Doing this now will only serve to escalate the situation further, and will result in the patient's needs being neglected.

D & E & F - While one can fairly state that these options have a good rationale behind them as at some point you should present your case and reasoning to your seniors and maybe the patient, your immediate concern should be to diffuse the situation and ensure that the patient is attended to. Furthermore, it would not be wise to discuss your reasoning with your seniors without having first assessed the patient to establish that the patient is well and the rash is not a significant issue.

G - This has not been selected as an appropriate first step as the correct options serve to address the needs of the situation in a more effective and appropriate manner. It is best to address the needs of the situation (apologise for your mistake, communicate why the patient was not reviewed and review the patient) rather than making the issue more complicated by trying to get the FY2 involved at the first instant.

Question 26: Doctor, She's turned red

This scenario assesses the junior doctor's ability to recognise their mistakes, understand their limitations, seek appropriate advice where indicated, and prioritise tasks.

The correct answers to this scenario are: **E.F.G.**

E - Phone the on-call medical registrar and get his opinion

F - Apologise to the patient for the mistake

G - Place the patient on evening handover to ensure that she does not deteriorate

E - Despite the fact that this is a surgical patient and you are a surgical house officer, the problem is a medical problem and the best person to seek advice from is the medical registrar on-call; especially as allergic reactions have the potential to become very serious and thus it is important to act promptly.

F - This is very important, and demonstrates probity. It is also essential for the doctor-patient relationship. The Good Medical Practice clearly states the steps to take when apologising to patients who have suffered harm or distress (paragraph 30).

G - This is another wise decision as there is a chance that there can be further complications. Thus it would be beneficial if your evening colleague casts an eye over the patient to ensure she remains well.

A - This is important, however, only after establishing that the patient is well and there are no other issues or complications. As the rash has just come on, it is a bit premature to offer this reassurance just yet.

B - Very basic clinical judgement will lead you to understand that the patient has suffered from an allergic reaction and not acute anaphylaxis. One cannot rule out that the reaction will not progress to anaphylaxis, however, commencing emergency management of acute anaphylaxis from the current level of information provided will be a significant overreaction.

C - This is not your first priority given the new developments. It is important the patient is safe from an allergic reaction before you think about alternative analgesia.

D - Same as option C.

H - This does not help any of the acute needs that have arisen in this scenario, and is not usually performed in circumstances such as this.

Question 27: The rush to discharge

Medical assessment units are very busy and the turnover rate is very high. If a patient is medically fit and ready for discharge, then ideally the discharge should happen quickly to make a bed available for the next patient.

However, unwell patients are always the priority. The nurse may be under pressure for beds, but it is the doctor's responsibility to ensure that the unwell patient is adequately assessed and is on the correct management plan. It is also important to note that the patient with hypertension also needs to be reviewed to ensure that he or she does not have any specific problem causing the high blood pressure. There may be other causes for the high blood pressure aside from not receiving the anti-hypertensive medication.

This scenario highlights many competencies of a junior doctor including: prioritising unwell patients, ensuring patient safety, working and communicating within a team and recognising one's own limitations.

The GMC's guidance states that *'you must provide a good standard of practice and care. If you assess, diagnose or treat patients, you must:*

a adequately assess the patient's conditions, taking account of their history (including the symptoms and psychological, spiritual, social and cultural factors), their views and values; where necessary, examine the patient

b promptly provide or arrange suitable advice, investigations or treatment where necessary

c refer a patient to another practitioner when this serves the patient's needs.' (Good Medical Practice, paragraph 15).

The correct answers to this scenario are: **A.F.H.**

A - Explain to the nurse that you won't be able to do her discharge summary as the other patient is more of a priority

F - Ask the SHO on-call to help you

H - Handover both patients to the night team

A - The unwell patient is the main priority and must be attended to first. Furthermore, the nurse may not have realised that the patient is spiking a temperature and requires urgent review.

F - If the on-call SHO is not busy with another patient, it would be advisable for them to review one patient while you review the other. This would result in both patients being reviewed as soon as possible. This option demonstrates that you have recognised your limitations, not in clinical competence but rather in the time limitations.

H - This is an important option as it is unlikely that you will be able to complete all the needs of both patients in 15 minutes, thus ensuring that the night team are made aware of the patients is essential. Both will most probably require input after any assessment that is done in the next 15 minutes, the unwell patient for further review and the patient with high blood pressure for completion of the discharge summary or further investigations if the high blood pressure is worrying. Do note that the option does not state that the patients are handed over at the expense of being reviewed.

D - It is expected for foundation doctors to be able to prioritise their tasks, especially in a situation like this where there is an unwell patient waiting to be reviewed. Thus, calling your senior to ask what to do in this situation is not favourable.

E - This compromises patient safety as the discharge summary is not the most urgent priority and the patient with hypertension also needs reviewing.

B - The unwell patient has to be fully reviewed, examined, investigated and discussed, it is not sufficient to simply ensure that they are on antibiotics and fluids. Secondly, the patient with high blood pressure needs to be reviewed too before discharge.

C - The importance of handover has been discussed, so, unless one is confronted by a situation where one cannot make the meeting due to the acute needs of an unwell patient, the handover meeting should not be missed. It is vital for the continuity of care and without it the new team will not be well equipped to prioritise their activities.

G - This is not appropriate for this situation, the best option would be to communicate your concerns to the sister in charge at a later time if required, especially as you are tight on time anyway. You also need to appreciate the pressures on the nursing staff to make beds available.

Question 28: No harm in exaggerating?

This is a very delicate situation that requires careful handling. When a senior colleague requests an action that you know to be incorrect, it can be very difficult to go against their wishes, and even harder still to highlight their mistake to them. Despite this, fundamental principles of Good Medical Practice should be applied here - that of probity and good clinical care. One must also demonstrate respect for colleagues, even in cases of disagreement.

The correct answers to this scenario are:

B.C.D.

B - Refuse to write details that are untrue and say that you will speak directly to the radiologist and try to persuade him/her to perform the scan today

C - Tell your SHO you do not feel comfortable writing details that are not true on the form

D - Ask your registrar what the best course of action to take is

B - Any radiology requests that are deemed urgent should be discussed with a radiologist. In doing so, they are prioritised according to their clinical need. It may well be that after discussing with a radiologist, the CT chest scan will be done on the same day. If it is not done on the same day, then the consultant should be informed as to why the radiologist cannot perform it that day. It is not within your capabilities to determine when patients are scanned.

C - As an FY1 doctor you will find that the majority of your work is done in conjunction with your SHO. This is a very close working relationship that relies on trust and mutual respect. It is important that the SHO is informed that you disagree with her advice, but this must be done in a polite manner. The GMC state that:

'You must work collaboratively with colleagues, respecting their skills and contributions.

You must treat colleagues fairly and with respect.

You must be aware of how your behaviour may influence others within and outside the team.'

(Good Medical Practice, paragraphs 35-37).

By telling your SHO that you feel uncomfortable as opposed to launching a personal attack, you would remind her of the importance of being honest in her work. Furthermore, prioritising your patient using false information could mean other patients in greater need of the CT scan are forced to wait.

D - The registrar is an important port of call when you find yourself unable to come to an agreement with your SHO. It is important, however, not to be seen to be undermining your SHO, and so a conversation between all three team members would be the most effective way to decide on an appropriate course of action.

E - The seniority and experience of your SHO does not mean her every decision should be adhered to, particularly when it is evident that the decision is unethical.

F - A stepwise approach must be taken when discussing issues with seniors. It would not be correct to approach your consultant directly without first attempting to discuss the matter with your SHO and registrar. However, should a resolution not be reached and you have concerns about your team that can not be resolved, it would be feasible to have a discussion with your consultant about your concerns.

G - Although this action would appear to absolve the junior of responsibility in this situation, this is not strictly true. As a doctor you have a duty to inform colleagues when their actions are contradicting best medical practice guidelines and potentially affecting other patients adversely, as is the case here. This must be done delicately as explained above. Furthermore, standing idly by as a colleague makes a mistake may well be seen, by the colleague, as a tacit approval of her actions.

H - This response is unsatisfactory as the action still involves dishonesty and the potential for harm to other patients. The resolution to ensure scans are ordered promptly in future would be a rational learning point from this scenario.

Question 29: Jehovah's Witness and blood transfusions

This scenario assesses the junior doctor's ability to understand issues pertaining to mental capacity, respecting patient's wishes and being pragmatic.

As has already been explained, consent is required for all medical interventions. All patients are deemed to have mental capacity unless it has been proven otherwise. Mental Capacity Act (2005) states that for a person to have capacity they must be able to:

- Understand the information being provided
- Retain the information provided long enough to be able to make a decision
- Weigh-up the information available to make a decision
- Communicate their decision (not necessarily verbally)

The GMC states: *'you must treat patients as individuals and respect their dignity and privacy. You must treat patients fairly and with respect whatever their life choices and beliefs.* (Good Medical Practice, paragraphs 47 & 48). Further guidance also specifically addresses the central issue of this case – *'You should not make assumptions about the decisions that a Jehovah's Witness patient might make about treatment with blood or blood products. You should ask for and respect their views and answer their questions honestly and to the best of your ability.' (GMC Personal Beliefs and Medical Practice, paragraph 11).*

'Group and Save' is when a sample of blood is taken for the laboratory to analyse so that in the event blood is required, the laboratory knows what type of blood to provide for the patient. 'Cross match' is when a specified amount of blood products are requested from the laboratory, for this you would have already done a 'group and save' or if not, you will need to send a new sample of blood for testing.

The correct answers to this scenario are:

A.D.G.

A - Accept the patient's wishes and document it in the notes

D - Do a 'group and save' in case the patient changes her mind

G - Refer the case to the medical registrar and ask him to help deal with the situation

A - Both respecting the patient's wishes and documenting clearly are vital in this case.

D - Patients can, and at times do, change their minds even in situations such as these, so it would be pragmatic to have the blood ready should the patient decide later that she will accept a blood transfusion.

G - It is vital to get senior involvement early in a 'life or death' situation such as this.

B - This is not a valid option as while you should clearly communicate the potential consequences of her action, it is not correct that you start persuading her to have the transfusion. The GMC state that *'you must not express your personal beliefs (including political, religious and moral beliefs) to patients in ways that exploit their vulnerability or are likely to cause them distress.' (Good Medical Practice, paragraph 54).*

C - This option is not permitted as has been explained above.

E - This option does not address the immediate needs of the situation.

F - This is a reasonable option and would be a logical next step, however, options A, D and G address the urgent needs of the situation more comprehensively and thus have been preferred.

H - Similar to option B.

Question 30: Compulsory FY1 teaching dilemma

As a junior doctor you will be constantly juggling different duties. This scenario depicts a common scenario where the team is not fully staffed - it is common not to have a full team as some members may be 'on-call' / 'on nights' / on annual leave / study leave etc.. Compulsory teaching sessions are vital to the junior doctor's professional development, and attendance is not based upon how busy one is, as if that were the case, many junior doctors would miss an innumerable number of sessions. At many trusts, attendance is monitored and has a bearing on the FY1's end of year assessment. It is important to note that teaching and training are also very important for patient care. This scenario tests the junior doctor's ability to prioritise tasks and work well within a team.

The correct answers to this scenario are: **A.D.E.**

A - Explain that your session is compulsory and you really need to go

D - Inform the Foundation Programme Director of this problem

E - Call the education department and seek their advice

A - This is the best option here as it is important that you communicate clearly to your senior the compulsory nature of the teaching session. It addresses the most immediate needs of the scenario. A one hour teaching session should not significantly impede your jobs, even on 'a busy ward'. It is important to note that patients who are acutely unwell will always take priority over all other needs and tasks, however, this is not the case here.

D - This action is advisable in this case because this problem has arisen three times now and the foundation programme director is responsible for facilitating your learning needs.

E - This is also a very reasonable choice due to your difficult situation and the conflicting demands being placed upon you. The medical education department may intervene on your behalf and talk to the registrar. Furthermore, they would be made aware of the reason of your absence should you not be able to attended the session.

B - This option takes a very passive approach, and while it may be true that not much can be done now, you need to take active steps to address this ongoing problem.

C - This disregards the registrar completely, especially when the team has additional pressures upon it, and is an unprofessional approach to adopt, even if you have legitimate reasons for leaving.

F - This is similar to option C, however, here you will receive little benefit from the teaching session by attending half way through.

G - This option does not address the heart of the problem and it is not a viable long-term solution, if adopted it will lead to a significant negative impact on your professional development.

H - This is incorrect, as one has to understand the registrar's perspective in this case, the demand he is making is not necessarily 'unfair' in the given context. There is a staffing issue and that has to be addressed.

Printed in Great Britain
by Amazon